BEAUTY
NOW WE'RE FORTY

MAGGI RUSSELL, forty-one, has been a writer
and editor for twenty years. Author of *The
Complete Book of Natural Beauty*, she has
divided her career between publishing,
health and showbusiness articles,
interviewing many major celebrities for
women's magazines. She currently lives in
Brighton and is studying for an English
Literature degree at Sussex University. Maggi
and Tina have been close friends for twenty
years.

TINA BOWLES, forty-one, spent the decade of
the seventies as Beauty Editor and feature
writer for *Honey* magazine. As a freelance
journalist she has contributed to a wide
variety of women's magazines, including
*Options, New Woman, Woman, Woman's
Realm*, and *Woman's Weekly*. She is
currently living in Tunbridge Wells and has
recently turned her attention to fiction.

BEAUTY

NOW WE'RE FORTY

Maggi Russell and
Tina Bowles

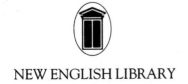

NEW ENGLISH LIBRARY

British Library Cataloguing in Publication Data

Russell, Maggi
  Beauty now we're forty.
  I. Title II. Bowles, Tina
  646.70082

  ISBN 0-450-51070-0

Published by New English Library,
a hardcover imprint of Hodder and Stoughton,
a division of Hodder and Stoughton Ltd,
Mill Road, Dunton Green, Sevenoaks, Kent TN13 2YA
Editorial Office: 47 Bedford Square, London WC1B 3DP

Designed by Behram Kapadia
Photoset by Litho Link Ltd, Welshpool, Wales.
Printed in Great Britain by Butler & Tanner Ltd, Frome and London

Contents

Night Cream · Eye Creams · Facial Exercises · Blemish
Busters · Moles · Hands · Feet · The Body Beautiful

Instant Giveaways · How to Fake Flawless Skin · The Eyes
Have It · Blush · Lipstick · Fingertip Control · Bare-Faced
Effrontery

Step by Step to Successful Surgery · Collagen Injections ·
Face-Lift · Eyelids · Noses · Breasts · Tummy Tuck ·
Liposuction

How a Body Ages · Fat Facts · Exercise · A Balanced
Diet · Your Body Type · How to Diet · Devise Your Own
Diet · Diet Saboteurs and Saviours · Detoxifying Diets ·
Slimming Pills · Vegetarianism · Vitamin and Mineral
Supplements · Your Exercise Routine · The Most Effective
Programme for Fortysomethings

To our sons, Edward and James

Acknowledgments

We would like to thank all the professional men and women who so generously gave of their time to contribute to this book, in particular Susan Fox of The Harley Medical Centre, Pauline Smart and John Terry of the National Hospital for Aesthetic Plastic Surgery, Dr David Fenton of St Thomas's Hospital, London, Dr Richard Horton of *The Lancet*, John Firmage of The Institute of Trichologists, Daniel Galvin and Mary Lou. And a special thank you to all our friends, who dispensed wit, wisdom and moral support whenever it was needed.

ONE

The Looks Crisis

'Beauty is an *experience*, nothing else. It is not a fixed pattern or an
arrangement of features. It is something *felt*.'
D. H. Lawrence, *Essays*

———————

'This is what forty looks like.'
(*Gloria Steinem* on being complimented on not looking her age.)

———————

What does forty look like? What *should* forty like? However you want it to. There is no one 'ideal' way of looking forty, and no one woman who embodies it. Nobody would compare Joan Collins with Anita Roddick, for example – both look terrific in their own individual, uncompromising way. If your looks don't toe the party line, don't panic – your way is probably still the best way for you. Perhaps you just need to develop your own personal style more fully or take a positive approach to health and fitness. This book is all about sailing through the forty barrier feeling good about yourself and looking better than ever. We hope that *Beauty Now We're Forty* will help you to do this in the same way that writing it has helped us.

What then is all this fuss about being forty? Forty is the age when you feel that you should still be looking young, but deep down inside fear that you don't. Sometimes you find yourself overcome with a strange longing to be fifty instead – because at least then you'd be *entitled* to have a few wrinkles without the accompanying guilt and shame. Forty can be difficult because it's a twilight zone – a transition between youth and fully fledged mature womanhood. Almost everyone has a rocky passage – you can't rely on the old way of looking good any more and yet you don't feel ready to try for something new. Carving out a new identity takes confidence, initiative and verve.

People don't like forty because it sounds so prosaic. Forty can seem to be the stuff of jokey birthday cards and cartoon books. But just because poets don't write odes entitled 'On Her Being Forty', and movie directors have not yet made the film called *All This and Forty Too*, or *And God Created Forty-Year-Olds* doesn't mean that they shouldn't be made. Much as you may be convinced to the contrary, people passing you in the street don't slide their eyes away to their shoes, whispering to each other, 'She's *forty* you know.'

In fact there's never been a better time to be forty. Look around you – so many of the most interesting and attractive women, whether they are writers, broadcasters, actresses or politicians, are now over forty. We have so much on our side now, and the opportunities are there in abundance. Women are no longer relegated to background supporting roles, and older women are acknowledged as having the very most to offer.

But these are early days. It is, after all, only in the last forty years that women have ceased to be regarded as only valuable for their biological function. Feminism has a toehold but there's still much work to be done – it really is up to every one of us to help shape its path.

Of course there will be times when we feel nervous and fearful about the future because we really don't know what we can expect. We know what we don't want: we don't want to grow old in anything like the same way as our mothers' generation did. But what will we replace this with? These are exciting times because we all have a chance to rewrite the script.

It's time to change. To change the way we view ourselves and the way the rest of society views us. Change is scary because it always involves the loss of something – in this case the safe old way of growing older. But change is exhilarating too because it can lead to self-mastery, personal power and an opportunity to redefine yourself. There is a lot to feel confident about, much to look forward to. But first we have to deal with . . .

AGE PANIC

Age panic hits us around our fortieth birthdays with the sudden realisation that time is running out; we are terrified that our looks, which we have relied on all our life, are waning fast.

Age panic begins in the mirror, but ends a million miles away. Of course the first wrinkles and grey hairs are depressing but the jolt they bring can have positive spin-offs. They remind us how far along the road we have already come; they tell us how far we have yet to go. At forty, we can look back on the past from a high vantage point and see the pattern of our lives emerge. From this we can gain insights into our personalities that were never available before. What kind of relationship do we form? How do we treat other people and how do we allow them to treat us? What kind of work inspires us and what kind has the reverse effect? Have we lived too recklessly – or in a narrow, timid way?

Best of all, at forty we have the luxury of time on our side. We can, if we choose, retrain or re-educate ourselves and still have the prospect of long working lives in our chosen fields ahead. We can pick up the threads of careers interrupted by marriage and babies and go on to achieve all we promised ourselves we would when we were in our twenties. It could be five or ten years before the menopause begins so technically there may still be several fertile years to go. Is this the right time to embark on family life? Or are there other, equally rewarding ways in which a need to care for and nurture others can be fulfilled?

'Forty' has that ring to it simply because our parents' generation always instilled that fear in us – to them forty was over the hill. They didn't have the opportunities, the health care or the beauty technology to look and feel as good as we do now. Our forty is more like their thirty. And it's very likely that by the time we're sixty we'll still be behaving like women in their forties. If we can muster the courage to grasp the nettle forty really can be just the beginning . . .

TEN TOUGH QUESTIONS YOU MUST ASK YOURSELF NOW

1. Have you got lazy? Do you put as much energy as you used to into your looks, your work, your relationships? Or do you exhaust yourself trying to be superwoman, controlling everything? It's time to loosen your grip – learn how to relax, share, delegate. Ruthlessly cut out dead wood. Spend the time you save lavishing care and attention on yourself for a change.

2. Are you indulging in self-defeating behaviour? Not bothering about yourself because you're too weighed down by self-pity? You must take responsibility for your own life from now on; it's too precious to leave in the hands of others.

3. Is your sex life as good as it could be? Do you *have* a sex life? Have you given up on it because you don't want to take risks or because you fear rejection? 'No time', 'Too tired' – are these just excuses? Sex is energising because it releases tension and boosts self-confidence.

4. Do you take your partner for granted? Have you forgotten what attracted you to him in the first place? He's an individual – not just your other half. Rekindle your friendship, devote some time to making him feel loved and wanted and the chances are he will repay your attention so that life for both of you will be enriched.

5. Are you feeling scarred by disappointments – have you been changed by the unhappy things that have happened to you? You can and must shake them off. Even bad experiences can be turned to good if we can learn something from them.

6. Are you still harbouring childhood conflicts? A longing for the kind of love that your parents never gave you can stop you loving yourself enough in adult life. This can manifest itself in all kinds of ways in adulthood: overeating, smoking, drinking heavily – these are all destructive comfort habits. It's time to rid yourself of emotional junk from the past. It's no longer of any use to you.

7. Are you more of a mother than an individual? Do you opt for motherhood to give you an identity because it's easier than going out there and making it as a powerful individual? Of course your children need you, but they don't need a doormat or a martyr. Aim to strike a balance which also allows you opportunities for self-expression and development, and this will benefit everyone. Children grow up quickly. Cherish the time you spend with them, but remember that one day they will leave home to start a life of their own. Where will that leave you if you've built your entire world around them?

8. Do you think you're nothing without a man? Many women feel anguished and empty without a man to take care of them. Needing love is normal and natural but you shouldn't feel worthless and desperate without it. Men don't go looking for a woman to take care of – they are attracted to strong, giving individuals.

9. Do you fear the unknown? Are you scared to change because things will no longer be familiar and safe? Change is always uncomfortable at first because you have to adapt your whole life to new modes of behaviour. But remember – no pain, no gain. And the ultimate reward of change is the *end* of pain.

10. Do you allow the rest of the world to walk all over you? Life today is tough. It's a jungle. No one offers you anything on a plate; you have to go out and get it for yourself. No one is going to help you, you're on your own. Deciding to be a beautiful, exceptional forty-plus woman could be the most frightening thing you've ever had to do in your life. It means being different. It means getting noticed, standing up for yourself and refusing to be ignored. It's the challenge of a lifetime.

WHY LOOKS STILL COUNT

Because our lives are so full of desperately important issues – money worries, caring for children, trying to keep marriages going, struggling through divorce, fighting for our position at work with a younger workforce biting at our heels – we tend to think looks are a superficial matter and the least of our problems. But this really isn't so. Your looks are your packaging – they are the only way the rest of the world has of telling instantly how you're doing, how you see yourself, what you're looking for and what their chances are of getting to know you better.

A woman who is beautifully groomed, elegantly dressed, confident and relaxed and fit-looking is obviously a winner. She cares a lot about herself – and as others always take you at your own self-evaluation, self-esteem in a woman shows that there must be a lot there to feel proud about.

Looking good is a love and sex issue, a career issue, a friendship issue, and of course a health issue. Perhaps this last is the most important of all, because if you are fit and strong, you can cope with the rest of life's problems far more easily.

FIVE AGEING MYTHS EXPLODED

1. Women go off sex as they get older. Not true! Surveys show that forty-somethings are more responsive, more interested in sex and generally much happier with their love lives than younger women. More relaxed attitudes and better, more honest relationships with partners are the key.

2. Men never make passes at women over forty. This is nonsense too. Many men prefer older women, but see them as unattainable. Or you could be putting them off with your dowdy, self-defeated air.

3. Older men only want younger women. Only certain kinds of men do – the ones who can only cope with women as inferiors. Young women give blind uncritical devotion, rather like pets. Older women want to be treated as equals. It really is better to wait for the right man than try to change the wrong one.

4. Struggling to look young is a depressing and losing battle. Not so. You owe it to yourself to look your best for as long as possible. How far you feel you need to go, with cosmetic surgery for example, is up to you. But trying to look good is not a sign of desperation, it's a sign of self-esteem.

5. *It's impossible to reverse the physical effects of ageing.* In fact everything – your skin, hair, figure and all round fitness – can be vastly improved by taking more care of yourself and seeking out the right treatments.

IT'S TIME TO TAKE ACTION NOW

We now know so much. We know how the right foods and exercise can give our bodies the best possible chance of ticking over healthily through the decades to come. We have new and exciting discoveries like Retin-A (a cream which, it is claimed, can reverse sun damage to skin) and minoxodil (a stimulant to hair growth). These undoubtedly will pave the way for more research aimed at alleviating some of the most depressing and socially alienating aspects of growing older. We have plastic surgery too. Plastic surgery has been dubbed 'scarification', and in one way of course it is; but many women find it also brings them increased self-confidence and a new lease of life – in other words, all the things we are warned not to hope for. How you view plastic surgery is a personal matter but no one can deny that it's *there*, increasingly popular, and that the stigma has been removed.

Radical feminists tend to dismiss beauty routines as shallow, frivolous or self-obsessed, designed to foster insecurity and thus boost consumerism. The reality is different. Caring about one's appearance is nothing new. The first skin cream was concocted nearly two thousand years ago, long before films, TV, glossy magazines and the advertising industry. Men and women have always devoted time to pampering and improving themselves, and the very act of doing so is in itself a therapeutic one. Grooming rituals provide a pause in the daily clamour of life and give us a chance to get back to basics, to get back in touch with our bodies. Life is so fast, so mechanical, so cerebral these days that we need to remind ourselves from time to time that we are, after all, human beings with blood in our veins. It doesn't matter whether it's a ten-minute soak in a scented bath, a brisk walk in the fresh air, or thirty seconds spent massaging in a moisturing cream, time spent beautifying and improving ourselves is precious time, time spent in peace and privacy, time spent on self-love.

When people are depressed one of the first things that happens is that they stop caring about the way they look. We now know that by helping someone to take pride in her appearance again we can actually help her to get better. It can be a starting point, a launch pad – a valuable aid to self-confidence and increased feelings of self-worth.

Beauty Now We're Forty is not about replacing youthful insecurities with a new batch of age-obsessed ones. No one is suggesting that from now on you must spend hours in front of the mirror, primping and preening, hell-bent on self-examination. No one is suggesting that you should spend even one minute trying to recapture your youth. It's a hopeless task. Nothing you do will really make you look *younger*. Not even a face-lift. But there are many things you can do which will make you look better, healthier, happier.

It's no good just heading straight back to the old routines. You've changed and you're going to go on changing. It's time to learn new skills and look at yourself from a fresh perspective. Use the confidence and self-knowledge that comes with age to enhance and enjoy your individuality. Don't waste any more time or money trying to match yourself to an impossible ideal.

Sorting out your appearance, getting back on good terms with your skin, hair and body, will release you to get on with the rest of your life with confidence renewed, morale sky-high. It is not the end of your quest for a fuller and more satisfying life. It is just the beginning . . .

TWO

Don't Doubt Your Sex Appeal

'Nothing is more ageing than giving up sex.'

'I never look at women under thirty-five,' swears Paul, a cuddly, bearded writer in his early fifties, loved by many. 'And women in their forties, if they take good care of their bodies, are the sexiest of all. There's nothing more erotic than undressing a well-groomed, sophisticated woman, and discovering a vulnerable femininity underneath. And the more powerful the woman, in personality or career, the more exciting this contrast becomes. I reckon it takes most women until their forties to *grow into* their femaleness. Young women are often boringly shallow and vain – even when they seem uninhibited they don't really have a clue how to enjoy a man's body. Sex is something that gets done *to* them. Older women are far more basic, urgent and unselfconscious about sex – they know how to give and take pleasure, and they don't fake. And a body that has given birth is a truly sexual body, not a turn-off at all. But I'm often saddened by how insecure older women are.'

Please don't pester us for Paul's phone number in a mistaken belief that this man is unique. There really are many more out there who feel just the same.

Perhaps Paul's feminine ideal would be a mature Marilyn Monroe, sharply suited and sitting on the board at Universal Studios, or at home in the bosom of her grown-up family. A heady combination of sweetness, maturity and power. Alas, Marilyn too lacked that essential faith in her own female worth.

Looking around for womanly archetypes in the media, we don't find them advertising such luxuries as clothes, perfume, alcohol or chocolates. The girls in these pictures are almost always under twenty-five. We then start to assume that if the forty-plus woman is rejected as a suitable image by media notorious for using sex to sell their wares then it must be simply because men don't fancy us any more.

And let's face it, *men* really are right at the heart of why we worry so much about looking older. The reason that most of us are scared witless by the crunch of heavy boots on the gravel, coming to march us away to our fortieth-birthday celebrations, is not because we are envisioning a desperate future of aching joints, hot flushes and strange hairs growing out of our chins, but because we're convinced we've lost our previous ability to drive men wild with desire. The more alluring you were at twenty or thirty, the more you will have come to rely on this talent as a reason for getting out of bed in the morning – especially if you were rash enough to bypass personality development for an obsession with firming up your inner thigh. (The truly smart girl, of course, dedicated herself to both.)

In a world without men, passing forty would give none of us more than just a moment's pause. If we were locked up *Tenko* style, with just our own sex for company, it would soon become apparent that the older, more experienced females were the most admired and valued members of the community. Silky blond curls would count for nought (except to a minority for whom *Tenko* features strongly in their private fantasies anyway).

In the real world, however, life is more complicated – and it's teeming with men. Male approval is what we seek – and why not? A *soupçon* of a sexual frisson here and there increases the adrenaline and adds some spice to humdrum life. If we deny that we have sexual power, or are too scared to use it in case we meet with rejection, then we run the risk of becoming lonely, cranky women, old before our time, and alienated from the seemingly sex-obsessed world at large. And with *every* sex manual telling us that far from being in decline, we are now mentally, emotionally *and* physically at our sexual peak, this would be a terrible waste of what could be – *should be* – the most exciting years of our lives.

Of course we're going to find current media ideals demoralising. Society still holds out the image of the nubile young woman as the reward for powerful men. It was Monroe who summed it up by saying that a young woman being pretty was the equivalent of a man being rich. One asset can be traded off against the other. And it's cold comfort to reflect that it was our generation who did most of all to foster the *totally modern* myth that only the young can be beautiful. The sixties was a time of the most appalling ageism. Previous generations weren't nearly so unenlightened. In the past, famous beauties, courtesans and mistresses of kings, were adored and admired well past their forties. Full-bodied, strong-willed women, their maturity was a major element of their appeal. Wisdom, wit and artful sensuality ensured they saw off their more youthful competitors and won the hearts of men, both young and old. Even in our mothers' day it was stars like Greta Garbo, Mae West, Marlene Dietrich, Joan Crawford and Bette Davis who held sway. These were Real Women, not simpering nymphets.

The current media ideal looks and behaves more like a twelve-year-old boy – breastless, hipless and lean as a gymnast. A body that photographs aesthetically in the nude, without looking too vulgar. So where do we fit in? We who should be settling nicely into the voluptuous prime of our lives, but instead are more likely to be found at home, gazing nervously into the mirror and doubting our ability to compete with the younger woman . . . when really there's no need for competition at all.

OLDER MEN – YOUNGER WOMEN

'The trouble with most women over forty,' says Jack, who is always happy to explore such topics, especially with a female audience over dinner, 'is that somewhere down the line you've allowed somebody to seriously demoralise you. And it's not men, you know, but *advertising men* who have done this to you. The worse they can make you feel, the more of their stuff you're going to buy. Nobody admits that women get more desirable and more interesting as they get older, because that would make them much too powerful. Men like young flesh because it's easier to dominate, not because it's firmer. Older women could have it all, but instead of getting out there and taking your pick, you're all at home alone, on the phone to your girlfriends, snarling about what bastards we all are.'

Small wonder. Take Jack for instance: why, if we're so fab, was he, a rich, handsome and divorced property developer of forty-five, going about with a mere snip of a girl of twenty-four?

Uneasy silence. 'Because,' he said finally, 'she doesn't put any pressure on me. I don't want to marry, move in with or make future plans with *anyone* right now. And I don't feel like being Uncle Jack to someone else's kids. I've been too busy having my own mid-life crisis to deal with anyone else's, and I did enough analysing with my ex-wife to last me a lifetime. Susie is fun – she rides horses, shoots, plays pool and knows about money markets, and of course she's very pretty. Who wouldn't enjoy such company?'

There is, of course, another side of this story. According to Cathy, who knows a thing or two about both of them, 'Susie is showing all the signs of a girl in the grip of a terminal obsession. She *worships* Jack, but is terrified to mention the Big C.' (Commitment, not the other.) 'She touched on it briefly once, and he showed immediate signs of going off her. Their lives are an endless whirl of gallery openings, cocktail parties and weekend breaks in posh country houses. This may be just a little interlude for Jack, but for Susie it's her reason for breathing. All she really wants to do is wander hand in hand round Sainsbury's picking up tasty snacks for two, and if he helped her choose wallpaper she'd die of rapture.'

The big joke is that grown-up women like us are far less likely to try to pin Jack's shiny wings to a board than Susie is. We've sorted our careers, had all the kids we want and been through most permutations of the male/female dilemmas. Now all we want is some light-hearted fun. And we'd have sussed out that that was all Jack was after, on the first date. When Susie hits twenty-six, she's going to start thinking about thirty – and wistfully picturing Jack behind a double buggy. When that time comes, Jack will almost certainly go back to his own wife and family, or find someone else to start all over again with.

There are plenty of men who really believe you are as young as the woman you feel. The pioneering heart surgeon Christiaan Barnard is a typical example. He is proud to have exchanged an older wife for a babe in her early twenties.

He's emphatic about why he doesn't want a wife his own age.

'I've always loved youth,' he told the *Daily Express*. 'I feel supremely happy walking down the street with a beautiful young woman on my arm, attracting all the attention. It makes other men jealous, and women furious,' he gloats. It seems he's given up heart transplants for the more exacting and lucrative science of trying to manufacture a successful anti-wrinkle cream. I only hope it works, for his wife's sake: otherwise some anxious moments, mirrorwise, are in her future.

Not all men are like this, but you'll find lots in certain high-profile, overpaid professions, where staying young is essential to staying on top. Most likely to succumb are those men who've grown up with a shallow set of values, low self-esteem and a desperate need for attention and approval from the outside world. If you're unlucky enough to be married to a man like this, he may well desert you for a younger woman when the mid-life crisis strikes. You can try offering sympathy and reassurance and the opportunity to talk it through. You can try injecting some excitement into your relationship with exotic holidays, sexy underwear and the gamut of sexual positions. But if none of this makes the slightest difference, you've probably little choice but to wave him and his toupee goodbye. This kind of man will never resolve his menopausal problems until he can make peace with himself. Don't waste time envying his girlfriend – she's got years of his agonising and angst ahead of her, *and* the unenviable burden of making him feel younger for ever. Instead heave a sigh of relief, shed a tear or two of regret and then set about the more rewarding business of rebuilding your own life on much firmer foundations.

Most of us will have to cope with a man going through the mid-life crisis at some point in our lives. Men worry just as much about losing their looks, and probably more. They also worry about their virility, or lack of it, and premature ejaculation, too. Thus jogging, vitamin pills and chasing young girls can become an obsession after forty.

They sometimes have affairs with their young secretaries simply because these girls are single, available and *there*. 'I was looking for a catharsis,' as one errant forty-five-year-old romantically put it, 'and if it hadn't been Sharon, it would have been someone else.'

Be kind if you can, for in most cases this phase will pass. Unlike us, who express our fears to anyone patient enough to listen, men bottle everything up or resort to drink. If he's your husband or lover, try not to seem too terrific yourself for a while. Don't laugh at him, or describe his situation in the most scathing terms (tempting though it may be). Don't pinpoint his past failures, harp on about where he's gone wrong, or immerse yourself in your own life and career to the point where he feels like a dispensable spare part. Be positive and supportive, as you would with a close girlfriend going through troubled times. Between you, think of ways to widen your horizons, improve your lifestyle and catch up on some of the things you regret you didn't do when you were in your twenties and thirties. If you're lucky life will become more stimulating, more fun and you'll be immensely grateful you have a partner to share it with who's wise, mature and knows you well. Many couples do work through this sticky patch and emerge closer and happier than ever before.

Meanwhile don't let the spectre of the younger woman haunt your every waking moment. There's nothing wrong with *you*, it's just that some men can't see the wood for the trees.

Ask most men if they prefer twenty-year-olds or forty-year-olds and a glazed look will come over their eyes. 'I'm sorry, but I'm not equipped to answer that straightforwardly,' replied John, to cross-questioning. 'We men have little sensitivity, no talent for introspection and negligible self-control. And we never discuss our feelings. How on earth can we be expected to know what women we really like? Generally we prefer *anyone* who won't give us a hard time. No man is rashly going to state that he prefers twenty-year-olds because he's canny enough to know that this is a blatant revelation of his own inner ageing paranoia. We like to think, though, that we can absorb youth by osmosis, preferably by pressing up against some sweet young thing. The reason a man leaves his perfectly adorable forty-year-old wife for his twenty-year-old secretary or co-star is not because he can't stand looking at her wrinkly face one more morning. It's because he wants to look into a pair of female eyes and see himself reflected as this shit-hot virile guy. Not old George, whose every failing is as familiar to you as the contents of the laundry basket.'

Men who have played the field, and lived life in the fast lane throughout their twenties and thirties, are likely to be far less confused. Take James for example. Attractive, unmarried and forty years old, he's devoted his life to building up his business, and has got through a string of girlfriends on the way.

'Young women are great to look at,' says James, knowing that with his looks, money and blemish-free past he could take his pick, 'but what on earth do you talk to them about? I was chatting to a twenty-three-year-old the other day about music, and happened to mention James Taylor. "Who's James Taylor?" she said. OK, that sounds petty and hardly a reason to knock a potential relationship on the head, but as far as I'm concerned it's a symbol of all the huge areas of my life and past that someone so young couldn't hope to understand or share, no matter how intelligent and sensitive she was. Young people are a different generation; they come from another planet.

'I don't need a pretty girl on my arm as a status symbol, I've got plenty of those already. And I don't need her to tell me I've done well – I know I have! No, I'm looking for a soul-mate now, a best friend, someone whose opinions I respect because I know she's developed them over years of experience.

'OK, I am a bit jaded now. I can't get excited about the same sort of things I got excited about when I was in my twenties. I think I'd come over as a bit depressing to a wide-eyed slip of a thing, on the threshold of life. I need to move on to the next stage, and of course I want someone of my own kind of age to help me through. Sure, I still want to have a good time, enjoy life, travel and all that, but I want to do it with people I have something in common with. And there are lots of things I don't want to do any more. I'm certainly not interested in hanging about trendy places just to be seen – that kind of thing. Neither do I want to feel there's pressure on me to behave like a sexual stud.

'I don't want to be anyone's idol, I want someone I can learn and take from, just as much as she can from me. And it's marvellous when I meet grown-up, attractive, confident women who can make *me* laugh for a change!'

FEAR OF THE FABULOUS FORTY-YEAR-OLD

There's a strong argument for the theory that many men, and particularly media men, prefer to try to ignore the forty-plus woman because actually she scares him to death. Sexiness needs to be coupled with a degree of submissiveness for the average male to be able to cope, and the image of the woman who is sexy, powerful, mature and independent is too alarming for words. We suspect that the continuing popularity of ladies such as Joan Collins and Elizabeth Taylor is because they display a great deal of vulnerability in their private lives, suffering deeply at the hands of men. Jane Fonda is remembered wistfully as Barbarella, not the paragon of politics and fitness she has become.

Men may admire the sexy, dynamic career woman of today, but they prefer it if she's married to someone else. Having spent forty years escaping the all-powerful mother's clutches, they don't want a replacement who will boss them about all over again (although they do, of course, want to continue to be mothered, but that's another thing). Of course truly wonderful, secure men marry career women and adore their grey cells as much as their pink ones, but whenever such a desirable, single Harrison Ford type pokes his nose out of his burrow and into the sunshine, he is immediately snapped up by a passing lioness who will take him home and guard him tooth and claw.

This paradoxical male view, this cock-up between the hearts and minds of men, was revealed to us over and over again in the confused statements men made about the women they admire and the ones they actually end up with. Thus many men who say older women are the pinnacle of feminine fulfilment, in reality avoid them like the plague.

Take for example this piece of whimsy from the famous photographer of celebrated beauties, Terry O'Neil who was asked to compile a list of the world's most beautiful women for *Woman* magazine. 'I think you have to mature in years before true beauty develops. The Princess of Wales is attractive, but she's too young – her personality hasn't really developed, so that inner beauty is missing. The women on my list are nearly all over forty. They have something special and it's not just physical beauty. In almost every case they have either a sense of humour, dedication, a loving maternal instinct or sheer professionalism, but they also look terrific. The difference is that these women look good without make-up and they're not dedicated to presenting an image. Most of them are very insecure and not the slightest bit vain – they blush when you compliment them, and that's a very attractive quality.'

Great stuff, you may think, here's a man worth his salt. But as one scans his list the heart sinks – no powerful women here, no natural beauties radiating sex and positive thinking, not one who can honestly be said to be more gorgeous now than she was at twenty, when each was considered the embodiment of female perfection. Not one escaped the trap of her own beauty – which meant she was used as a commodity, and loved and left in droves by men. As a result, one is dead of a drug overdose, another is a recluse with her cats, face ravaged by too much sunbathing, another is only a tentatively reformed drunk, and yet another only recently restored from a bloated, drug-addicted wreck. It is their blushing vulnerability our photographer is attracted to, not true beauty which stems from self-esteem and control over one's destiny. To cap it all, this very same admirer of the mature female split from his very powerful, beautiful middle-aged wife to live for a while with a model just out of her teens. We rest our case.

So what is the sexy, powerful, forty-plus but single woman to do? She wants a lover her own age, and she doesn't want to hide her light under a bushel to get one. And if she doesn't find a man who appreciates her soon, she's going to start imagining it's because she's this wrinkled old prune of a woman with cellulite and a spongy stomach – not a madonna worshipped from afar at all.

Of course many women in their forties have devoted husbands who love them better as the years go by, and others have toy boys tucked up at home waiting impatiently for them to rush home from the office. They have problems too – but more of that anon.

THE YOUNGER WOMAN AND YOU

An alarming number of our friends – attractive, successful, kind-hearted women – through no fault of their own, find themselves alone. Re-entering the mating arena after years of marriage and motherhood is the hardest step of all – how the rules have changed! In the sixties we were submissive dollies, waiting for men to call, dreaming of being picked up in Jaguars and taken to rock concerts, while we ironed our hair, shortened our skirts, and practised that knock-kneed Jean Shrimpton gait. Naive and sweet was the order of the day.

In the seventies and eighties we firmed up our acts, realising that if we weren't going to marry Mick Jagger we'd need a career. We lost interest in the seething morass of males for a while, contentedly raising our kids, pursuing our dreams, marrying men without a clue what our futures would bring.

Suddenly it's the nineties and the world has gone all strange. Girls are wearing mini-skirts again – but now it's an act of aggression. They sneer at the snapshots of our soppy young selves, limp-haired, soft-thighed and shabbily attired. Young women today are spiky and lean, cool and tough – and if they're not, they're hiding at home, trying to develop anorexia and Madonna's insolent stare. Clothes have become so skimpy only girls built like Michael Jackson can wear them.

There seem to be a depressingly large number of these about. Indeed surveys show that women really are getting taller, thinner and stronger. They are starting to look more like men.

Men our own age are both fascinated and disconcerted by this image of the modern Ms. Used to subtlety and secret stocking tops, they are amazed by these girls who wear their bras over their jumpers and suspenders below their hems. The modern girl, in turn, is not at all uninterested in the older male, boys her own age being much less openly impressed with her charms. Who at any age would not prefer a cuddly, craggy male with money and manners to a boy you have to fight with to see in the dressing-table mirror?

So what is your stance in the battle for these few, endangered creatures: desirable men, mature in experience and years? Of course you may eschew them in favour of younger men, in which case your life will take a different course. Or you may feel more like Pamela: forty-one, divorced, manageress of an up-and-coming furniture chain and mother of a seven-year-old son. 'I just don't feel sexy any more: and I suppose that's why I'm convinced I'm not. Men don't look at me in the street like they used to, and quite frankly I don't blame them. I scurry along looking tense and worried, with no make-up on because I haven't had time . . . I have a full-time job which is mentally very demanding – not chosen because I'm graspingly ambitious, but because I need the money that goes with it to maintain a normal, decent lifestyle for my son and myself. But the net result is that I'm completely knackered most of the time. Vulnerable? Feminine? Hah! Here I am earning the money, running the house, maintaining the car, looking after my son, with some part-time gardening thrown in – I feel more like a haggard, harassed Super Woman. I know I don't need a man to survive, I can manage just about everything on my own, but as a result I've lost touch with the side of me that responds to men. As a sexual being I simply don't know myself very well any more.'

DO YOU HAVE A SENSUAL SELF-IMAGE?
So, you've been too busy with your family, your career and your financial problems to pay much attention to the way you look or feel. It's definitely time to take yourself in hand.

Elsewhere in this book we'll be telling you everything you need to know about making your outer body as beautiful as it can possibly be. This is the time to talk about the inner you. The part of you where you *feel* sexy, desirable and female – at least you would if only you allowed yourself the luxury. So much of your energy has been going into other people over the last ten years, you've probably forgotten that divine introspection that you indulged in at twenty, that vibrant self-awareness that made you feel like the sexiest women who ever walked the earth. And all you had to do was close your eyes and fantasise . . .

While young women habitually meditate on the erotic side of life, we, out of sheer exhaustion, are in danger, whenever we close our eyes, of drifting off into the great blue nirvana where being has no form. This is not the answer. We are used to male admiration and lust – we've grown rather attached to it, and we're not ready to give it up. So instead of concentrating on a mantra that leaves you an empty vessel ready to be filled with spiritual calm, it would be better to lie on the sofa thinking filthy thoughts which stir you into a lather. You are what you think.

Why don't men sidle up to you in the street any more, whispering endearments? Why don't strangers rub against you when you're strap-hanging on the train, grown men grovel at your feet, cars crash into each other as you pass?

Because you didn't spend two hours getting dressed and made up this morning, just to go and hang out at the local joint, looking for men. Because you are not wearing the following 'come and get me' gear: bright red lipstick, stilettos, tight mini-skirt, midriff-baring T-shirt, jeans ripped in strategic places to show red suspenders underneath. In other words you no longer look like an easy lay. Of course very young girls with totally flat bodies can get away with this, as demonstrated in fashion magazines, because they look innocent and boyish enough not to know what their clothes are saying. As soon as you add the wobble factor – a real, womanly bosom and hips – these clothes start to look unspeakably rude. Men love this, but women will spit at you as you pass.

Your working schedule probably allows you something nearer ten minutes for getting dressed every morning, and the demands of your day dictate clothes that are functional and safe. Clothes that will take you to the office or the supermarket usually show serious intent. Men do not respond to these clothes – so they do not see you. But although you are no longer giving off blatant sexual signals, occasionally a man may glance at you. Oh my God, you think, is my blouse gaping open? Have I got pigeon-shit on my head?

No – it could simply be that the real, sensual you has shone briefly through, like a ray of sun from behind the clouds. Just because your sexual antennae have withered away and fallen off, just because you can't tell now when a man really fancies you, it doesn't mean that they don't. Just because you're paranoid, it doesn't mean that they're not still out to get you.

Of course, you know that your days of attracting random, marauding men are over. Unless of course you want them back, then all you have to do is revise your wardrobe a little. Just think what a hooker might wear, put it all on and go and stand on the corner of your street. A dangerous traffic situation will develop around you in minutes.

Alternatively, you might like just a few, selective men to acknowledge your existence as you pass. To do this you will have to retain certain items of feminine attire in your daily costume. They can be subtle and tasteful, but still convey that basic message – that you are a sensual women.

When in doubt about any aspect of your wardrobe, just ask yourself, 'Would Jacqueline Bisset wear this?' If the answer is a resoundng no, hasten the item Oxfamwards with ne'er a backward glance.

CHILDBIRTH, YOUR BODY AND YOUR BRAIN

Just as men are at the crux of whether you worry about your age or not, childbirth is at the root of how you feel about your body. Regardless of the fact that your body may have scarcely altered at all, your brain perceives things very differently. Mother Nature, domineering matriarch that she is, has seen to it that you no longer regard your flesh as solely designed for the pleasure of men, but as a means of nurturing your children. And your brain no longer sees thinking up new ways to entertain your lovers as its prime responsibility, but instead selects nest-building and worrying about little Joey's rashes as your major concerns. Before you know it, your sensual self-image has been completely destroyed, and instead you see yourself as a lap and six arms.

Hot on the heels of the total demise of fancying yourself comes the conviction that all men must find you repulsive, too. You begin to exaggerate wildly about your peculiar-shaped breasts, your stretch marks that glow in the dark, your sponge-pudding bum, and the stomach folds that the cat gets lost in.

It's time to get back a sense of proportion.

WHAT MEN REALLY THINK ABOUT THE MATERNAL BODY

By the age of forty most of us have had one or more children, and our bodies are different from how they were at twenty. Many of us are actually leaner, fitter and altogether shapelier, with puppy fat and spots all long gone. Others of us have undeniably let ourselves go through the pressures of hectic or too-boring lives. A beautiful body can be regained at any age – and so can a good body image.

Paul, who has had many lovers over forty, is emphatic that their bodies are barely different from young girls' at all, and the ways in which they are different can be very attractive. But these women are so critical of themselves, they rarely believe anything he says.

Men do not expect to undress a mature woman and find her body to be just like a seventeen-year-old's. It would be most disconcerting if it were – a bit like undressing Robert Redford and finding Michael Jackson inside. Many men are *more* turned on by the look of the mature female body. One photographer told us how he is fascinated by silvery stretch marks, particularly if they're highlighted by a golden tan; another man told us how soft flesh is very welcoming and fuller figures are greatly loved, and one man muttered hoarsely about the droop of a heavy bosom driving him crazy – before having to excuse himself to go and lie down for a while. Your body shows your experiences as your face shows your character, and your individuality is at the root of your appeal.

Alex, a very stylish, silvery-haired advertising executive of forty-nine, only fancies much older women. In fact, at a bare forty-odd, *you'd be much too young for him.* 'I find older women very exciting and always have done,' he says. 'I'm attracted to them mentally and physically. I like them to be well-groomed with stylish hair, well-manicured nails, expensive clothes. I like buxom women, not skinny. Simone Signoret – now there's my idea of a powerfully sexy woman. Although I'm married I have long love affairs with older women. Some women, when I meet them, haven't had sex for years. They're like sleeping beauties, and it really excites me to wake them up.'

WHAT'S SEXY	WHAT'S NOT
Shrugging off physical flaws	Agonising after perfection
Admitting your age	Pretending to be younger
Blushing as a man undresses you	Doing a striptease
Showing him the real you	Wearing make-up all night
Mussing up an immaculate woman	Staying perfect no matter what
Being too plump	Being too thin
Serious lace and elastic underwear	Cotton Calvin Kleins

WHAT'S SEXY	WHAT'S NOT
A glimpse of scented cleavage	Dresses slashed to the waist
Dancing all night	Aerobics all day
Seeing the funny side	Sarcasm

HOW TO MAKE LOVE TO YOURSELF

When we were younger, we lay around the house fantasising about men and sex all the time. Now, lying around the house is an unheard-of luxury – and if we do it, it's because we've got the flu. Next time you have a spare ten minutes, resist the urge to grab the biscuit tin and tune in to *Neighbours*. It's time to rediscover licentious things.

SEXY THINGS TO DO

Take slow, perfumed baths
Read the *Story of O*
Massage your body with aromatic unguents (not green gritty gunk supposed to melt cellulite)
Wear silk pyjamas
Lie on your bed in nothing but silk stockings and then . . . masturbate.

How you go about this last item is desperately important. Of course you know *how* to do it – so we won't embarrass you with lurid talk or that ghastly text-book jargon about masturbating being good for you to maintain elasticity and lubricity as if you were some mechanical inner tube. We're talking about your most alluring, feminine and mystical parts here. And of course you are an expert on what gets you off. But if this should be something bizarre to do with football teams, vicars or policemen with truncheons, why not try a different tack occasionally? Focus on your own body and how magically erotic it is, the mystery of your inner organs, the blood in your veins, the silky velvet quality of your insides, the sheer glory of your voluptuous womanly flesh. This will plug you into a state of oneness with the great goddess Gaia, or at least get you finished and off to sleep in thirty seconds flat.

HOW TO MAKE LOVE TO A MAN AT FORTY

The same way you did at twenty, except try to do it with twice the passion. Nothing, not tensile nipples or double-jointed hips, is more exciting than good old-fashioned enthusiasm.

HOW TO MAKE LOVE TO YOUR HUSBAND OF TWENTY YEARS

The same way as to a husband of twenty minutes. You've just got lazy, that's all. According to one sex therapist we're hardly ever too tired for sex – we just think we are, that's all. Sex doesn't sap energy, it actually releases physical and mental tension, so you'll feel refreshed and renewed afterwards, not tired and drained. Next time he has a headache, seduce him. Give him the works. Sex for its own sake will cheer you up and calm you down. It takes you back to basics – it reaffirms life, and it's a much more interesting way of doing your pelvic floor exercises. Let your imagination run riot, both in what you do and what you think while you're doing it. According to this same sex therapist high libido people usually have the most vivid sexual imaginations.

BANISH BRAINWASHING
Most of us are seriously brainwashed women – convinced that because our bodies do not embody the golden section, no man who wasn't desperate could really want to take us to bed. From this moment on, you must completely cease from reading the following kind of magazine articles. Just go cold-turkey on them right now.

How to completely alter your legs in three weeks. (Only a bad accident can do this.)

How to judge if you have drooping breasts by suspending pencils under them. (Your breasts deserve more respect.)

Nazi-style thigh-fascism that exhorts you to exterminate your cellulite.

Exercise routines that involve bashing your bum against the wall.

Photographs of six foot, thin, straight-nosed, full-lipped, golden-maned athletic models. (Many men prefer plump, big-nosed brunettes, honest.)

Slimming features with before and after pictures where the 'before' pictures look just like you, and the 'after' look just like Glenys Kinnock.

Fashion spreads showing clothes designed by famous homosexuals, which make no concessions to hips or bosoms, because these men want to make women look like boys so they can live out their fantasies of cross-dressing without getting arrested.

THINGS WE KNOW ABOUT MEN NOW WE'RE FORTY
When we were twenty we were attracted to aggressive, sexy, domineering men, the adventurers, dreamers and schemers of this world. Many of us are gratefully divorced from one of these now, unable to tolerate the constant infidelity, egocentricity and inability to fix the broken cutlery drawer that goes with this kind of man, because he is too busy on his private designs for an alternative Channel tunnel. Now that we no longer get our excitement solely from men, but create our own, the more companionable kind of man is tops. Now we stay away from beautiful men – gods are not our type. Do we want to be constantly clearing away the debris left by other women who fall at his feet? No, sirree. Give us a short, bald, kindly sweetheart any time, who hasn't allowed the pursuit of muscle definition to stunt his personality. Of course saying that all handsome men are bastards is just as sexist as

saying that all beautiful women are dumb – but it's almost impossible to be gorgeous and not be vain. And vain is a pain when you live in its shadow.

Some men who have it all – looks, power, money – are unhappily very contemptuous of women. These are the ones who go out with bimbos, to whom they're unspeakably rude. Get one of these men between the sheets and you find out why – sexually, he's meagrely endowed. Not used to failure, they like to be the ones to do the rejecting – so don't take them on unless sex therapy is your forte.

Men are not really turned off by fat women. They just let us think so to keep us in our place. Many men, not just the inhabitants of Tonga, are seriously turned on by copious female flesh. The big woman embodies everything female – devouring and comforting, demanding and loving. Dr Loring Chapman, Professor of Psychology at the University of California, is convinced that by the twenty-first century, fat will be fabulous again. In the meantime you could do worse than take a holiday in Egypt. One journalist friend of ours, forty-eight, blonde and a statuesque size eighteen, has just returned from a trip down the Nile, ecstatic about the reception she received. 'They were like moths round a flame,' she crowed. 'Egyptian men are marvellous, and they simply worship, big, beautiful women of a certain age. For two weeks I felt like a goddess!'

While we don't see this as an excuse to bury our noses in the trough after twenty years of dieting, it's something to think about next time you feel a flesh flagellation session coming on. And looking around at the women you know – isn't it weird how all the fattest ones have devoted husbands?

Men, like pasta, come in all sorts of quirky shapes and forms, and there *are* Nice Men out there somewhere. Oh yes, there are – except they rarely live in inner cities and they *never* go to cocktail bars. Well, our friend Jenny claims to have met one once, but she can't be sure because they were both drunk at the time and he must have lost her phone number.

Nice men are *never* famous artists who have blue periods, rock stars who croon of honky-tonk women, or writers who go to hookers claiming it was just in the interests of research. And they never work in the film industry. (Except David Puttnam, maybe.) Nice men, if they're not at home with the wife and kids, are busily committed to meaningful, low-paid careers, or perfecting some ancient, long-forgotten craft for which there is little call in today's mercenary world. So you are unlikely to meet one in flashy watering holes. However, he may call round to fit your kitchen or landscape your garden, so be on the look-out all the time.

Another name for the Nice Man is the New Man. Unhappily, he has become somewhat unfashionable of late, dismissed as wet, unsexy and something of a wimp. He had a brief spell in the limelight in the late seventies, before a fiercer financial market and various social psychologists decided that men really are genetically designed to behave like bastards after all. To illustrate their point they directed us towards the behaviour of male gorillas, assuring us that we are all still primates at heart. Thus all the aggression, competitiveness, promiscuity and egocentricity that goes into being considered one helluva bloke is just nature's call. We, meanwhile, remain unconvinced that modern man's less savoury qualities can be dismissed as secondary sex characteristics. Some men are simply nice, and some are not, just as we'd bet that there are plenty of sweet-natured gorillas who kiss good night on the doorstep, and send bananas round in the morning.

WHY WE DON'T WANT TOY BOYS

A recent survey by a hair colour manufacturer set out to discover just how much women over forty enjoy sex, and with whom. The results showed either that we are far sexier, more imaginative and orgasmic than ever before, or that some women, somewhere, have had a great laugh at the expense of some gullible interviewers. This is what they claimed: two-thirds say their sex lives are much better than when they were young, three-quarters have done it in the living room, the bath, the car and regularly on the kitchen table, and one in ten wasn't with her husband at the time.

Fourteen per cent of Londoners have affairs, 43 per cent have sex two or three times a week, 4 per cent every day. Fifty per cent choose lovers the same age, while only 4 per cent go for younger men. Nine out of ten don't want any more children, so sex is purely for pleasure.

Perhaps the 4 per cent who have sex every day are the same 4 per cent who have younger lovers. This, of course, is the great advantage of selecting them young. So what are the pros and cons of the younger man?

The Pros

'One of the lovely things about being forty today is the attitude of young men,' purrs feline actress Kate O'Mara, forty-nine. 'Joan Collins created a vogue for older women which reshaped my career. I dreaded my fortieth birthday, but now I feel, what have I got to lose? This gives me a tremendous feeling of freedom and confidence. Sex is much better now there is no longer the fear of getting pregnant. I look better than I did in my twenties. No longer soft and vulnerable, but sharper and tougher, which is more interesting, but I'm still the same shape and size.' Kate is quite open about the string of young lovers who trail after her, reeling with admiration.

It's definitely true that the older woman is a highly fashionable asset for a younger man – proof that he has the sophistication, class and style to keep up with her. He also has to have a high degree of self-confidence – Cher's young beau, scarcely half her age, hardly wavered by all accounts when she ordered that he should be 'stripped, washed and brought to my tent'. (Don't try this unless you have at least half her chutzpah or cash.)

Chrissie, aged forty-two, has two lovers of twenty-six and twenty-four. 'Sex with young men can be much more relaxed and humorous than with men my own age. But it's more tender, too, as they are not cynical, or set in their ways. They're capable of changing, and because they were brought up with feminism they understand what equality is all about. I have my own flat, car, and a high-powered job – but my boys don't find this threatening. They see me as a woman of substance who is far more of a challenge than a woman of their own age.'

The Cons

The reason that the older man/younger woman syndrome is more common than the other way round is not because we can't attract younger lovers so easily, but simply because we don't want to. Frances Lear, editor of the American magazine for older women *Lear's*, says, 'I don't need some boy who hasn't witnessed birth or death telling me that I'm wonderful.' Well, maybe some of us do, but we know deep down it's only going to be a temporary situation. Unless the young man in question is exceptionally mature, problems are bound to develop later.

Rachel finished a four-year relationship with a lover twelve years her junior because 'I found myself looking anxiously in every mirror I passed, to see how much I'd aged since the last time I looked. I always felt embarrassed in front of his friends – I knew they were very, very curious about me. My own friends were supportive, but I could see that none of them really thought he was for keeps. Stephen was very hurt when I broke it off, but I knew one day he was going to want kids, and my child-bearing years are definitely over.'

Of course many women do have children by a much younger man – and this gives the relationship a far greater chance of success. But unlike Britt Ekland, most of us don't have the time, money or energy to go back to Nappy Valley all over again. For a woman in her forties who positively *wants* a child, a young man can be a perfect choice, as most men in their forties have had all the kids they want, too.

But even Chrissie, riding the wave with her two virile young beaux, admits that she doesn't expect the situation to last for long. 'Young men are emotional babies really, and although you can bask in their adoration for a while, eventually they're going to mature, and probably go off with younger women, ready to take a more dominant role. They are avid to learn about sex, wine, food books and music – but once you've taught them all you know they will be casting around for new experiences. My family are very disapproving, and my lovers never mention theirs – so we're very much on our own. And I'd hate to drift on with a young man with no future plans – only to be left at sixty when he's barely past forty. Ideally I'm hoping to end up with a man of my own age. Till then, my boys help to pass the time very pleasantly!'

REASONS TO FEEL SEXY

But why, speaks up a small voice, why go on with all this Sturm und Drang sexual stuff; why not just chuck it all in and opt for a tranquil, stress- and germ-free existence, ignoring men for the pleasures of books, girlfriends and gardening? Is this really what God intended, that we go rampaging on, tussling in this undignified fashion until we're drawing our pensions?

What's the point? Isn't it all rather, well, unseemly? Yes, it is. This is what makes us interesting. Why have we got all this heightened sexual chemistry, these not infrequent urges?

It's to keep men and women interested in each other, that's why, not just for breeding children. Nothing is more ageing than giving up sex. Everything just dries up. Your hormones say, 'What's going on here – *nothing?* In that case we'll just close down the plant. There really isn't any point in going on.' Then everything – skin, hair, body shape – is affected.

Without sex, men and women would retreat into separate camps – women to grow strange things in pots (we never lose the urge for fecundity), men to the dogs. Not healthy for either. Sex keeps men at home, putting up natty little herb racks. Of course men *can* go on giving babies until they drop dead at ninety. So their urges must be met. And who are they going to be doing it with if not you? You're simply going to have to take on these silvery-haired old gents, because no one else will be able to find the bits of them that work. And you're certainly not going to be able to do that unless you've got some fantastically well-practised fantasy in your mind. The sexy never grow old, and that's that.

THREE

Finding Your Individual Style: Your Clothes

'Forty is the age for elegance, for drama and for style.'

WHY DO YOU DRESS THE WAY YOU DO?

It creeps up on you so slowly you hardly realise it's happening, but then one morning you wake up (usually shortly past your fortieth birthday) to find – bingo! your clothes have turned against you. All your old friends – the baggy sweaters, jeans, long skirts and shapeless jackets – suddenly look hopelessly scruffy and untogether. Your anxious, creased brow stares back at you from the mirror as your lips form that morbid question – 'Am I dressing *too young?*'

Before you panic completely and rush out to Aquascutum to stock up on various Thatcherite blue suits, support tights and ruffled blouses, hold tight. Your wardrobe may well be overdue for some subtle revising, but the situation is seldom as dire as you think. It *is* perfectly possible to wear Levi 501s until you start drawing your pension, as long as you do it in the right way. Only the tacky, the cheap and the shapeless must go. The young get away with monstrosities because the contrast between sleazy clothing and fresh young figures, or outsize menswear and frail little waifs, looks somehow witty or cute. Over forty it can look desperate or drear.

Forty is the age for elegance, for drama and for style. Settle for nothing less. You are going to find out what really suits you best, ignore fashions that do not flatter, buy less but spend more. It's time to bend your clothes to your will, build up a wardrobe you'll want to wear for ever, and throw out everything that screams out that you got stuck in a time warp back in 1975.

Down to basics. First a little test to see how you and your clothes are getting along together right now.

What are you wearing right this moment? Are your clothes:

A. *Perfectly suited* to whatever you are doing?

B. *Flattering,* comfortable and stylish?

C. *Your everyday personal best?*
If you can answer 'Yes!' to all three of these, you are either Paloma Picasso or Inès de la Fressange, and I'm very flattered that you are reading this book.

If, on the other hand, your clothes are:

A. *The first thing that you trod on* when you got out of bed this morning

B. *Shapeless,* baggy and body concealing

C. *Not what you'd like to be wearing* when your partner's wife/mistress/ ex calls round uninvited – then, like most of us, you need a serious confrontation with your wardrobe. Even highly paid and much discussed celebrities need to do this, as has been revealed by the sight of some of the appalling things they are caught wearing by snooping paparazzi who then betray them to the Sunday colour supplements.

Your clothes, if not controlled, will always betray you – they are walking advertisements for your personality and insecurities, and speak volumes about your moods. If you look as if you've taken a great deal of trouble, you're telling every passing Joe that you're desperate for approval. If you look as if you haven't bothered at all everyone knows you're down on your luck. Always wearing sweatpants is a sure sign of terminal depression, just as always wearing stilettos is a sign of terminal anxiety about your sex appeal.

Dressing right all the time seems too much to ask of anyone, especially your average harassed and beleaguered woman of today. If only you had nothing but the *right* clothes in your wardrobe – clothes that suit you, clothes that fit, clothes you can just fling on and feel okay, clothes that make you feel ready to crack a few jokes with Dorothy Parker or sing a duet with Tina Turner – then you wouldn't ever have the problems getting dressed in the morning that you have right now.

How did that state of affairs come about? Why is your wardrobe full of things that are drab, shapeless and way past their sell-by date? Why, no matter how much any woman has to spend, does she *still* never have enough clothes? Why, after the amount of time and money they cost you, do your clothes always seem to be out to do you down?

It's probably because you don't know how you want to look and you don't know how to shop. Over the famed temple at Delphi, some ancient but crafty high priestess (no doubt in Yves St Laurent white toga, gold sandals and matching arm bracelets) had carved into the stone the immortal words 'Know Thyself' and 'Nothing To Excess'. She probably pinched these pearls of wisdom from some *soigné* classical boutique, for no better advice for clothes shoppers could there be. Engrave these words upon your own heart, for they are the very essence of the perfectly wardrobed woman.

KNOW THYSELF

Since the Bible informed us 'And they sewed fig-leaves together and made themselves aprons' women have never had a thing to wear. Although we have progressed to closets that overfloweth with God's bounty, and no one in her right mind ever goes near an apron, we still don't feel enthusiastic about anything we own. This is because most of it was bought with someone else in mind. Pink looks great on the au pair, that dress with a cross-over back looked very sexy on a stranger, and Daphne from number 16 has this really nifty way of wearing hoop earrings and jungly print turbans with loose black linen dresses. We rush out and order up the same, only to look like an applicant for Mrs Mops. Think again. Who are you? Ignore *everything* that doesn't look as if the designer used you alone for his muse. Don't buy aqua blue just because it's there. Don't buy white because fashion writers say you must. Know the basic shapes and colours that suit you, and stick to them doggedly until death you do part.

NOTHING TO EXCESS

The essence of elegance for women over forty is definitely that less is more. Fashion has gone mad and flicking through *Vogue* for inspiration just taxes your biceps – looking at old copies we're struck by how ghastly a lot of clothes look just a few years on. Even revered names like Yves St Laurent go through unspeakably embarrassing lapses where they send unfortunate models out down the catwalks in tiger print dressed with green feather boleros, black stockings with white high heels, lurid clashing colours and all manner of fussy, frilly horrors that look as if they have been thrown together by a maniac on LSD let loose in a haberdashery department.

The outfits from the past that still look utterly cool, delectable and up-to-date are all the most simple shapes, beautifully cut and pure in colour, by designers such as Calvin Klein, Donna Karan and Ralph Lauren. The Americans have got the message – Nothing to Excess. No mixtures of purple, orange and lime green, no puffballs, trapezes, hot-pants or see-through. (Even the young are undoubtedly going to regret some of these, as Princess Anne so plangently pointed out in 1971. 'Hotpants are the limit,' she said. 'People complain you are not with it, but certain things I will not do.') Just think about how we cringe over the platform shoe, the A-line mini, the loon pants and those utterly nauseating knee-length white plastic boots with drawstrings at the top. Yes, we wore them once, even though we've long ago burned the evidence.

There is only one dimension where the 'nothing to excess' rule can be broken, and that is with jewellery. Ever since the first truly glamorous woman emerged, Ursula Andress-style, from some primeval swamp and immediately started adorning herself with stones, tusks, and mammoths' teeth, women and men have weighed down their limbs with baubles and beads, and hung things the size of saucepans from their ears – and still managed to look perfectly serious and sane. Humans are meant to wear jewellery and look oddly unfinished when naked without it – a few bangles and chains make a woman look fearless and fit for anything. Perhaps this is a kind of armour. Cleopatra and Boadicea knew this, and passed a few tips on style down the centuries to Elizabeth I and Coco Chanel. We predict that the breastplate will be back in a big way any day now – several continental designers have already tried to reintroduce it. Maggie Thatcher has just been measured up for hers.

God definitely intended us to wear his earth's bounty – why else do pearls, platinum, diamonds and emeralds suit a girl so well? But clothes are different. We don't believe God meant his creation to wear animal prints, skirts that puff out, 90 per cent of Christian Lacroix outfits or fluorescent pink cycling pants. He *did* mean us to wear anything flowing and soft, anything with a minimum of seams. Oh, and we do think he meant us to wear shoulderpads (only not in negligees like SueEllen).

YOUR CLOTHES AND YOUR BODY

Of course the most fundamental reason why you dress the way you do comes right down to whether or not you like your body. If you are tall and slim with curvy bust and hips, you match the cultural ideal so you've no right to moan and designers are falling over themselves to dress you. If you still don't look sexy and stylish then you must be a very perverse person and deeply masochistic to boot. For the other 99.9 per cent of us who are short, round, flat or wide in all the ideologically incorrect places, creating a personal style is harder work. We are fighting against a media that doesn't value us the way we are, and constantly exhorts us to try harder to change our shapes. Our culture is not now comfortable with feminine values, and women are at war with their bodies. Our greatest fear is looking fat in our clothes – we just *know* we look fat without them. We've come a long sad way from Marilyn Monroe in *Some Like It Hot*, described by Jack Lemmon as walking like 'jello on springs'. Men thought she was pulchritudinous beyond belief in that film – a female director would have been exhorting her to shed twenty pounds.

We all have our 'fat' clothes and our 'thin' clothes, the former being what we wear most of the time. But it's really time now to come out of the camouflage. With a bit of thought, it *is* possible to get into the swing of wearing things that cover *and* flatter, to enhance our curves rather than to negate them.

It is a fact of life that women who wear clothes they adore, rather than clothes that simply make them look thinner, are perceived as more attractive by the rest of the human race. If flame silk Zouave pants reveal the fact that you have forty-two-inch hips, so what? They look a damn sight more sensuous and appealing than the shapeless black sweatpants and huge baggy T-shirt that you hope disguise your avoirdupois, but actually shriek to the world that you've got something to hide.

Society as a whole is not going to change its taste until the mature, maternal woman is truly on top where she belongs. But until then, you *can* refuse to be underrated and ignored. It's time to swathe your body like a goddess, instead of trying to garb it like an adolescent boy. And if you think that's going a bit over the top, at least dress with your own body in mind and not Kylie Minogue's.

HOW TO DRESS THE WAY YOU REALLY WANT TO

'Style is knowing who you are, what you want to say, and not giving a damn,' said Gore Vidal. Of course we all know who we are, we're just a mite inhibited about expressing it, that's all. It comes down to that fruitless old fear of looking foolish, of not conforming, of non-acceptance by our peers. There are strict rules of appearance for grown-ups who want to get on in the world. Only the rebellious young are expected to dress weird and wacky to show that they have a healthy disrespect for the old values.

We have our uniforms for *every* aspect of our lives, mostly chosen for us by other people. Our children want us to look like Ma in *Little House on the Prairie*, our men want us to look like Marilyn Monroe in *Bus Stop*, and our bosses want us to look like Sigourney Weaver in *Working Girl*. Mostly we buckle down and try to comply, but there's still enough leeway for the real you to have her say.

If we truly didn't give a damn, and decided to dress from now on just for ourselves, what would we really wear? It might not come as a big surprise to find that overnight we'd all changed into clones of radical lesbian feminists. It could be boiler suits, dungarees, desert boots and cropped hair to a woman because – let's face it – at present, the main factor we take into consideration when getting dressed every morning is whether or not we ever want to have sex with a man again.

Sex is at the root of all female dressing. Women who still want sex have wardrobes full of ridiculous restrictive things – tight skirts, high heels, silk bustiers, strapless dresses. Women who are positive that they don't ever want to have sex again immediately disappear into Harris Tweed suits, polyester blouses and brogues. (Unless you are a reincarnation of Vita Sackville-West, in which case you probably look impossibly dashing in men's suits, hats, cravats and waistcoats, and have tempestuous affairs with Violet Trefusis types – or maybe you favour George Sand and her 'smoking'.)

Sex is everywhere – it permeates the air we breathe like carbon monoxide and cooking smells. As long as we still want to be part of it all, we have to add some sex appeal to all of our uniforms. Men can wear anything – baggy tracksuits, smelly trainers and even *anoraks* and still get laid. We, meanwhile, seem eternally condemned to sartorial schizophrenia: you may spend your day reconstructing the ozone layer or producing a workable theory to solve the Third World Debt but you've still got to do it in lace underwear, a Chanel suit and three-inch Charles Jourdans. That is, if you still want to be deemed a woman.

But enough carping. Dressing up can be great fun too, not to mention a morale booster and a self-indulgence, so if you've got to do it, you might as well do it with gusto. Refusing to participate just further depletes your armoury in the internecine strife between us and them.

The road back to sanity and living in peace with your clothes lies in the understanding that A. You have to wear uniforms, and B. You can still make them interestingly your own.

FINDING YOUR INDIVIDUAL STYLE TYPE

There are four basic style types that most people more or less fit into: Classic, Creative, Sexy and Free-Spirited. Most people stick fairly close to one of these categories all the time, others play about with different personas for different functions – but you have to have enormous wardrobe space and free time to do this.

Perhaps ideally we could dress Classic for work, Creative for leisure, Sexy with men, and Free-Spirited with our children. To avoid a massive identity crisis in your closet and a horrendous final confrontation with loan sharks, it would be better to settle for one basic wardrobe and just add items from another style type as an occasional experiment.

CLASSICS

Icons Princess Diana, Grace Kelly, Audrey Hepburn, Jackie Kennedy Onassis.

Acolytes Royalty, politicians, lawyers, aristocrats, estate agents.

Items and colours Cashmere sweaters, striped blouses, Chanel suits, Hermès scarves, pleated skirts, floral tea dresses, tweeds, twinsets, Mulberry trenchcoats, pie-frill necklines, hand-knitted sweaters with teddy-bears etc., taffeta ballgowns, Chanel bags, Gucci luggage, pale tights, pearls, hand-made shoes, family jewels. Navy, beige, red, cream.

Best of the look Riding boots, trenchcoats, pearls, luxurious sweaters and pretty print frocks.

Descriptive phrases 'Quiet good taste.' 'She's a class act.' 'How frightfully grand.'

Designers and shops Jaeger, Catherine Walker, Whistles, Edina Ronay, Wendy Dagworthy, Ralph Lauren, Margaret Howell, Russell and Bromley, Emmanuel.

Cheap end Laura Ashley, Next, Marks and Spencer.

What you're saying 'I'm elegant, ladylike, successful, rich – and I believe in the status quo.'

CREATIVES

Icons Diana Vreeland, Tina Chow, Paloma Picasso, Barbara Hulanicki.

Acolytes Advertising and media personnel, designers – anyone in anything visual.

Items and colours Black tights, great jackets, short or ankle-length black skirts, constant sunglasses, men's watches, Armani suits, big shoes (Doc Martens or Japanese), vast leather tote bags (containing filofax, camera, vodaphone, manuscripts, work-out gear, lunch), chinos, black leggings, Alaïa short tight dresses and suits, Calvin Klein underwear, designer belts, ethnic or crystal bracelets and earrings (all huge). Black and more black, taupe, brown, yellow, red.

Best of the look Bodysuits, shoulderpads, black leather, menswear shirts and jackets, outsize silver jewellery.

Descriptive phrases 'I picked up this jacket in Japan.' 'I blew a month's salary at Donna Karan.' 'The Katherine Hamnett collection was an absolute nightmare.'

Designers and shops Yamamoto, Issey Miyake, Armani, Alaïa, Gaultier, Galliano, Westwood, Donna Karan.

Cheap end Miss Selfridge, Warehouse, Wallis.

What you're saying 'I'm stylish, progressive, in with the in crowd and definitely going places.'

SEXY
Icons Cher, Joan Collins, Elizabeth Taylor, Britt Ekland.

Acolytes Sixties models, rock stars' wives, publicans' wives, croupiers, transvestites.

Items and colours Leather trousers, suede suits, leopard prints, cowboy boots, black or white denim, rhinestones, furs, slingbacks, Janet Reger underwear, sequin dresses, streaked hair, tans, short tight suits, lace, gold jewellery, diamanté, high heels, sunglasses, Estée Lauder perfumes or Joy by Jean Patou. Red, purple, black, white.

Best of the look High heels, satin bustiers, denim, cowboy boots.

Descriptive phrases 'She's still right tasty for her age.' 'I'd love to see what she looks like first thing in the morning without all that make-up.' 'What an old tart.'

Designers and shops Yves St Laurent, Rifat Ozbek, Butler and Wilson, Manolo Blahnik, Bruce Oldfield, Anthony Price.

Cheap end Oxford Street shops with names like 'Lisa' and 'Estelle', Indian-owned leather emporiums, continental boutiques, Sunday street markets.

What you're saying 'I like men, and I'm exciting, glamorous and extrovert.'

FREE SPIRITS
Icons Isadora Duncan, Mata Hari, Frida Kahlo, Vanessa Redgrave, Colette.

Acolytes Painters, poets, actresses, alternative therapists, earth mothers, antique dealers, dropped-out aristocrats.

Items and colours Black turtle-necks, hand-printed textiles, kimonos, hand-painted silks, ethnic embroidery and jewellery, antique silver belts, extraordinary brooches, rings and pendants made by friends, sarongs, Navajo sweaters and ponchos, turbans and strange hats, beaded slippers, Japanese ensembles that look like origami, palazzo pants, antique lace, vibrant scarves. Any bright colours, strong patterns, black.

Best of the look Sarongs, drapery, original jewellery, inspired colour combinations.

Descriptive phrases 'We've just got back from Goa/Bali/Tibet.' 'We're just old hippies.' 'In tune with the planet.'

Designers and shops Byblos, Ghost, Gallery of Antique Costumes and Textiles, Talisman Gallery, Liberty, Lunn Antiques.

Cheap end Markets, auctions, bazaars.

What you're saying 'I'm unusual, sensitive, other-worldly, spiritual, unique.'

DRESSING TO SUIT THE OCCASION
The truly well-dressed woman always has the right clothes for the right situation. Of course wearing totally the wrong thing will make you stand out from the crowd, and men may find you strangely endearing, but supercilious style-sheep will sneer at you and make you feel insecure. Better to put them in the shade with your complete at-oneness, both in appearance and attitude, with the matter in hand.

Here, then, are some indications of what looks good when.

At home Sweatshirts, jumpers, jeans, tunics and leggings, pyjamas, jumpsuits. *Avoid* Tracksuits, especially in velour. The tops look okay with jeans while the bottoms look passable with a long T-shirt, but together they make *everyone* look fat, dowdy and like a retired gym mistress.

Travelling Loose cotton layers and sandals in summer, woollen ones in winter. Comfortable shoes at all times, as feet swell. Long loose skirts are better than pants as they are cooler during all that sitting. *Avoid* Short tight skirts that wrinkle, boots, tights, jumpsuits that go all flat on the bottom and are hell to take off in aeroplane loos.

For working out Black footless tights and oversize T-shirt if you're overweight, leotard and tights in any colour if you're thin. The best trainers or jazz shoes you can afford, cotton socks. *Avoid* Tight things that reveal the bulges you're trying to get rid of, and whatever your figure, forget Flo-Jo in her white lace bodysuits or cropped tops and bikini pants – these will just make the rest of the class hiss at you behind your back.

At the beach All-in-one black swimsuit: try on *hundreds* until you find one with the right bust support and bottom coverage to suit you. Having found it, buy two or even three – you may never find such perfection again. Huge patterned cotton wraps – to wear round hips, knotted above bust or toga style with a belt. Leather thonged sandals – gold looks great. Straw sunhats, turbans to protect hair. Waterproof make-up and sunglasses. *Avoid* Swimsuits with skirts reminiscent of Princess Margaret; underwear looks in bikinis – in fact no bikinis at all; toplessness – neither elegant nor good for delicate skin.

For sex Anything unspeakably exciting involving satin, bones, lace, see-through, suspenders, seamed stockings, high heels. *Avoid* Red and black nylon ensembles, baby doll nighties, crutchlessness, black rubber unmentionables (be suspicious of the man who asks for these).

For depression Trenchcoat and dark glasses, pulled down felt hats, leather greatcoat (the first to make you feel as if you're starring in a Truffaut or Bergman movie, the second so people don't recognise you, the third as a kind of armour-plating). Oh, and definitely a huge terry-towelling bathrobe and fluffy slippers. *Avoid* Anything revealing cleavage, legs, neck. No heels, frills, jewellery or colour. You need to be able to hunch and huddle into your clothes.

For recovery Anything red, the colour of assertiveness and vigour.

For work Suits, coatdresses, dresses with matching jackets, blazers and tailored skirts, tunics over narrow skirts. Pick simply styled suits in neutral colours – mauve or yellow may look stunning but you and your co-workers will tire of it very quickly. The style needn't be too severe – look for curvy jackets, just-on-the-knee skirt lengths for straight skirts, long if they're full. Large contrasting buttons look stylish. Underneath, silk T-shirts, polo necks, wrapover shirt shapes. Opaque black tights, medium-heeled courts. Buy the best quality you can afford in natural fabrics, wool, tweed, flannel, velvet-collared pinstripe. Think *LA Law*. *Avoid* Short tight coquette suits, pale colours (except on the warmest days), anything that makes you look emotionally vulnerable or fragile. Uncomfortable high heels, bowties, clanking jewellery, mannish briefcases, tights that snag.

For parties Invest in a few fantastic frocks and wear them to death. Perhaps two long, two short, a beaded jacket and thirties-style black halter-top pyjamas would see you through most situations. Choose dark rich colours, flowing lines, strapless, lace sleeves, billowing skirts or fluid slender columns, plain colours, simple shapes, bustled at the back. Perfect examples: Valentino red silk strapless column, swathed and falling in pleats at the back; Dior brown satin with full skirt and heart-shaped bodice; plain black jersey, demure at the front, slashed to the waist at the back. Long gloves and long dangling earrings, hair up or very full. Look for luxurious fabrics: silk, satin, velvet, lace. Silk shoes. The little black dress is still unbeatable. *Avoid* Frilly, shiny, bright pink or aqua blue, ruching that looks like Austrian blinds, bouffant skirts and hair, feathers, sequins.

For dinner parties Think of Martha Graham dancewear – dresses with wrapped top, fluted bias-cut long skirts with suede high heels, sarong skirts, beaded tops. *Avoid* Too much cleavage (puts off other diners), bustiers if you get a roll of fat hanging over the back when you're sitting, short tight skirts that ride up, constricted waist.

TWENTY FASHION FAUX PAS THAT FORTY-PLUSSES MAKE

1. Wearing mini-skirts just because they looked good on you first time around. You may still have the legs but you don't have the face. There's something highly unnerving about the back not matching the front view – a bit like that moment when Norman Bates's mother turns round in the rocking-chair in *Psycho*. From the back you see a nice long-haired lady, from the front a dried-up corpse. We jest – but not much. Coltish legs below a mature face look as if your top has been matched with the wrong bottom in a kids' card game. If you've got great legs, wear sarongs (sensational in suede).

2. But don't totally eschew the trendy – up-to-date touches show you are in tune, culturally aware, still ready to boogie. Look for the latest ways of wearing jewellery, scarves, belts. Most of all, keep up with the latest shapes in shoes.

3. Don't get too smart – too rigid clothes, hairstyles that are sprayed stiff, severe tailoring are all very untouchable and ageing.

4. Don't buy cheap – it makes you look downtrodden after a certain age. Chain stores are fine for classic lines, or find some mid-price designers you adore. (Jean Muir or Nicole Farhi will never let you down.)

5. Don't dress too timid – tiny jewellery, cardigans and pleated skirts, sensible shoes, all make you look mousy.

6. Flat shoes can look frumpy but are necessary for hectic lifestyles. Wear heels as high as you can comfortably cope with for the life you lead.

7. Don't always wear things that match – it's too contrived. The bag, gloves, hat and shoes don't all have to be the same colour, perhaps bag and shoes in one colour, hat and gloves in another.

8. Avoid wearing entire outfits by one designer. This usually looks very overdressed. Try the Chanel jacket with your jeans, the Armani suit with a cheap white T-shirt.

9. Don't save things just because they're not worn out – some things are indelibly stamped with a certain year and then look very passé, such as Marks and Spencer cotton crewneck sweaters, stonewashed denim, blouson leather jackets.

10. Dress for yourself and your looks, not your age (so ignore item 1 about mini-skirts if you truly look great in them).

11. Never wear trousers too baggy or too tight. A visible panty line is the pits. Trousers should be full through the hips with soft pleats, and should fit snug at waist and crotch. From there the fullness should be along the outside of the leg, not between. They should skim the top of the foot in length, and fall easily without pulling across the top of the thighs, rear or stomach. Jeans should never look trouserish, so they shouldn't have straight loose legs – wear them close fitting but never so tight you have to lie down on the floor and do them up with a coat hanger.

12. Shorts are very dodgy; if you want to wear them on holiday, choose loose-legged, mid-thigh length, belted varieties, never tight or very short.

13. If you must wear animal prints, go for one hit only, with a chiffon scarf, belt or cuff. Think of Jackie Collins in all those leopardskins ensembles – need we say more?

14. Boycott young fashions even if you have the body for them. Cutaway bare midriff vests, cut-off jeans, transparent T-shirts over bras often look tacky even on the nubile.

15. Accentuate your breasts in subtler ways: wrapover tops that show a hint of cleavage, jackets and dresses with nipped-in waists, draped or deep V necklines.

16. Well-fitting underwear is essential. For big busts good support is a must. The cups should enclose the entire breast; overflow at the top and sides is instant death to your clothes. Choose pants cut high in the leg and snugly fitted at the waist: bikini pants give no support, and frills show ridges. Never wear underwear so tight that flesh bulges above or below, but a little lycra and elastane goes a long way to give hips a sleeker line.

17. Don't wear tights that are cheap, baggy, snagged, patterned or coloured 'American tan'. Opaque is best for day, sheer by night – and only in light colours if legs are flawless and unmarked. The new tights with lycra are a joy to wear, and stockings should always be long enough to avoid that poochy overhang of inner thigh (although men inexplicably quite like this).

18. Hats should only be worn for a reason, i.e. to keep your head warm or cool. Keeping hats on indoors is just too Lady Bracknell.

19. Leave witty items to the young – think how soppy Princess Diana looked in her deejays and bowties, and fancy-dress army uniforms. (We know she's not forty, but she might as well be for the life she leads.) And think of Pamela Stephenson in all those tiresome hats and trinkets.

20. Beware of sticking with colours that no longer suit you. It's easy to get in a rut with this – changes in skin and hair colour need a total reappraisal of your clothes. Consider going to a colour consultant (several advertise in *Vogue*); you don't have to take their advice as gospel, but experiments are likely to pay off well. Finding your right colours could be a revelation – others will say how well you look or enquire if you've just come back from holiday. A pale, pasty complexion becomes warm and and peachy next to the right shades, and sludgy eye colours become bright and true. All-one-colour dressing looks very stylish, such as chocolate brown, navy, grey or bottle green. All-black dressing either looks impressive or hellish –just follow your mood, bearing in mind that it accentuates everything.

Accessories 'In matters of grave importance, style, not sincerity, is the vital thing,' said Oscar Wilde, who certainly knew a thing or two about accessories, whether it be to unmentionable sexual acts or to purple velvet smoking jackets. Wallis Simpson understood this too, hence her penchant for her own Cartier-crafted crown jewels. For the rest of us who don't have a little kinglet to send backwards and forwards to Bond Street, the important point to remember about accessories is that there *is* no point to them at all unless they are unutterably stylish, and sincerity as in owning the bona fide real thing has little value here at all. Fake *can* be fabulous – and who needs to wear the equivalent of our national trade deficit clasped around her delicate little wrist when Butler and Wilson paste looks just as stunning?

Over forty, women and jewellery come into their own. Important pieces need confident, knowing bosoms to nestle upon, while sensational earrings look ill at ease framing faces that haven't seen a shocking sight or two. Likewise hats sit more happily on women in their prime, while younger heads should be tousled and free, and much older ones run the risk of looking much too hatty and batty. At forty you really can go a little mad above the ears, having the dignity and elegance to carry it off.

'Shoes,' says Mimi Ponds (a woman after our own hearts), 'are more exciting than sex, more powerful than money, more essential than men.' Leave the young to their Doc Martens, Japanese sandals and smelly trainers; eschew espadrilles, banish ballet slippers, condemn the clog. You are for supple suede court shoes, high-heeled patent shoes, sleek leather boots and slender sandals. And when you are feeling too exciting even to risk being seen out, slingbacks, ankle-straps and unspeakably naughty open toes. As Bette Midler says: 'Give a girl the right footwear and she can conquer the world.'

At this point in your life, attention to detail really counts. Psychologists swear that your watch reveals all the nuances of your character, while the wrong bag can put your back out for life. Some women have this damned clever knack with scarves, but they're almost always continentals – we don't seem to have progressed much since Auntie knitted that cute Rupert the Bear look for our fifth birthday. Over forty, the serape, the wrap, the *throw* is for you. (But do be wary of the *shawl*, the traditional prop in pantomine to show that a character is aged and fallen on hard times.)

Here, then, is a brief guide to making your accessories *l'embarras des richesses* rather than just plain embarrassing or akin to the tasteless excesses of the very rich.

SHOES

The right shoes, when spotted in shop windows, make your innards contract and your heart skip a beat. There are basically two kinds of women in this world: high-heeled ones and low-heeled ones. Decide which you want to be, and embrace your destiny. To help you make up your mind:

High-heeled women – Joan Collins, Dolly Parton, Birgit Nilsson, Sue Lawley, Tina Turner, Elizabeth Taylor, Victoria Principal.

Low-heeled women Meryl Streep, Audrey Hepburn, Katharine Hepburn, Diane Keaton, Mia Farrow, Julie Christie, Vanessa Redgrave.

In other words, high-heeled women use their bodies while low-heeled women use their brains. This is not to say you cannot be taken seriously and wear high heels. Sue Lawley, in our opinion, has achieved this. To be relentlessly low-heeled is to be lacking in a certain zest for living. The key is to match your heel height to the moment. The eighties will be remembered for the bizarre sight of women in sharp business suits and trainers, rushing to work to change into equally extreme high heels. They took to heart Monroe's pronouncement that 'It was the high heel that gave a big lift to my career.' While sex and power are undoubtedly brother and sister to the shoe, a modest heel height will see you through the worst work-day calamity with allure and arches intact. The rule here is low heels for every activity except sexual activity. Then the skyscraper's the limit. *Always* buy as expensively as you can – cheap shoes pinch, rub and fall apart where good shoes receive your foot with a loving embrace and are faithful for life. An investment such as crocodile Manolo Blahniks could well be bequeathed to your grandchildren.

Of course you all know the obvious ploys of matching your tights or stockings to the exact shade of your shoes to make legs look long and svelte, and not wearing ankle-straps if the words 'thick' or 'chunky' could even remotely be applied to your calves. Dark shoes are always more flattering than light ones (unless they're a fleshy beige), and nobody with any credibility wears white high heels.

When girding your feet for sex, remember that shoes have a fetishistic connotation in all societies, so the symbolism must run pretty deep. No time to analyse that here, but remember anything unspeakably kinky and rude is fine for parties and dinners at home with your lovers – i.e., anything that involves the words thongs, shiny, strappy, stiletto, fluffy or mulish in their description. But don't go out in these unless you want every conversation addressed to your feet, and you are just looking for an excuse to keep saying, 'Rise, sir, from this semi-recumbent posture.'

We could go on and on about shoes but won't – suffice it to say that *anything* that makes your feet look like they once belonged to Ginger Rogers (slender, shapely and elegant) should become a treasured part of your life, and anything that doesn't should be cut off immediately without a kopeck.

JEWELLERY

There are two types of women in this world (we promise this is the last outing for this phrase): those who wear jewellery, and those who do not. Whereas Maggi can honestly say she has never seen an earring that she considered too big, Tina never wears any jewellery at all except a friendship bracelet her son made at school. While we have talked long and hard into the night to determine why this should be, we have never come up with any satisfactory character analysis by way of explanation. Quiet people do wear big jewellery while loud ones wear none, so that is not the answer. Certainly arty and sexy people seem to wear more than more retiring types, and the rich definitely wear more than everyone else put together. Perhaps some people should wear less and some wear more, but the essence of successful jewellery wearing is that items should be few rather than many, big rather than small, and unusual rather than mass-produced. Real gold, silver or precious stones are a joy to wear, but less effective than a designer fake if the design is ugly or the piece too small.

Jewellery should really be art to wear – it's your chance to make your style unique, and it's much better to wear odd jewellery than odd clothes. The latter will get you laughed at, while the former is a guaranteed conversation opener. Jewellery has lots of personality. Start collecting pieces you love and you'll always have something to match your outfit, whether it be mock ivory and silver cuffs worn with black or white, or translucent milky pearls worn with a peach satin peignoir.

For the nineties, natural materials will be tops. Look for stone, ebony, wood, sharks' teeth and bone, and forget the precious stones in favour of quartz, amber and crystal. Large charm bracelets give you a chance to collect your favourite symbols and personal objects hung round the neck on silk cords pull a look together in a very individual way, whether it be Japanese netsuke or antique jewelled compacts and lockets. Bold and dramatic is the key, nothing delicate, hesitant or fussy.

If anybody wants to buy you something real, buy a collector's item. This means anything by Bulgari, Fulco di Verdura (the Chanel designer), Jean Schlumberger (for Schiaparelli) or Tiffany. Ex-Dior designer Isabel Canovas makes amazing pieces, such as brilliant green resin foliage brooches crawling with real gold snails – sounds vile but they're stunning and no one else is going to have one. Think rare, exclusive, witty, exquisite.

A final word about pearls: it's no coincidence that older women adore them. Worn near the face they impart something of their own creamy glow to the skin. Look for chokers and ropes with big glass clasps, and forget about pathetic little pearl ear studs in favour of big oval clip-ons.

WATCHES

Have you noticed how interesting people wear interesting watches? You can definitely find out all there is to know about a man by taking a quick peep up his sleeve. Anything with gold and diamonds on – avoid this tacky person like the plague. Anything with chronometers, deep-sea divers' gear, bullet proof and shock absorbent – this man has a serious macho problem. Mickey Mouse? He's probably got Donald Duck on his boxer shorts, too. Fob watch? Pompous old fart. Black, high-tech, digital gadgetry, maybe with four faces giving times in London, Paris, Tokyo and New York? Identity problems and an inability to express feelings. He doesn't wear one at all? You'll probably never see him again.

With your own watch, go for a classic style every time. Antique Rolexes and Cartiers are all beautiful, reliable, functional and stylish. A low-key watch shows maturity and self-confidence. Go for Piaget, Mappin & Webb, Omega, Tissot, Gucci, Patek Philippe, Tag-Heuer, Audemars Piguet Ebel or Baume & Mercier if you want to buy modern. Jewellery watches can work well, such as a Breguet antique peacock blue enamel, or crystal Van Cleef & Arpels, but they won't go with everything you wear.

Maggi has just two watches, a simple stainless steel fifties Rolex and a flat round gold Victorian watch picked up for £15 in a junk shop. Both go with everything, merge in with other jewellery and are all the time increasing in value. They are personal friends who don't intrude unless consulted, then give totally reliable information without fuss or show. What more could anyone want?

BAGS

Bags are a problem, we don't mind admitting. We really envy men who manage to cram everything into their pockets. Soppy little purses and clutches are too neurotic and feminine, while briefcases are far too butch. Handbags over the arm *à la mère* are too gruesome to mention, and vast pouchy things, while useful for hiding your bottom, are a serious hazard to your back. Health-conscious Americans wear theirs across the body, but you've got to look like a cheerleader to have even a remote chance of getting away with such gaucherie. Shoulder bags are essential as the hands must be kept free, but small shoulder bags such as those disgusting gilt and quilted Chanel things are too uptight to mention. And anyone who has initials on her bag that are not her own – you are too far-gone-consumer-crazy for redemption.

The answer still has to be briefcases for work and a high quality burgundy calf leather remains the most popular female choice. For leisure, a medium-sized pouchy or saddlebag shape in black or brown is the best choice, canvas holdalls are best for travel, and there's no escaping the clutch for going walkabout at parties like Princess Di. A slim envelope under the arm is the royal favourite, but you still have to keep one arm clamped to your side all night which limits one's capacity for spontaneity to say the least. Paloma Picasso makes beautiful little evening bags got up to look like books, but they're still a nuisance to carry. Some are very small and loop around the wrist – pretty, but they won't hold more than your keys and a lipstick. Until we are liberated enough to insist on pockets, even in the skimpiest evening dresses, we'll have to go on sacrificing comfort for a smooth body-line. Belt or 'bum' bags are right-on okay for casual wear, with jeans or tracksuits.

SCARVES

Being clever with scarves enables you to soften your whole silhouette, while adding colour, prints and style. Prints work much better in scarves than they do over a whole outfit – and sometimes the bigger and splashier the better. Top designers are brilliant with scarves: at collections they wrap them at neck, hips and round heads. English women still cling to the Hermès scarf as the epitome of good taste, but Liberty prints are much more stylish and individual. There is a fine line between wearing a scarf brilliantly around head or hips and looking like an extra from *The Voyage of Sinbad*. If in doubt, stick to the neck and shoulder regions, but wear your scarves bigger, *over* not under your collar, and in the best fabrics and prints you can find. On the beach, a large scarf is indispensable as a sarong-style cover-up for self-conscious thighs. It's worth experimenting here as nothing adds such instant style, while covering up a multitude of sins.

HATS

Hats can look like fancy dress very easily – even the royals make many mistakes here. They can look charming, whimsical, individual or silly, eccentric or downright mad. Of course mad ladies can show off mad hats to perfection: think of Vita Sackville-West or Edith Sitwell in her turbans. Hats sum up an era more than any other dress item – think of those fifties petal hats to show what little flowers women really were, and Jackie Kennedy in her perky little pillboxes. Our favourites are romantic wide brims as worn by Restoration ladies, but we always feel overdressed when wearing them. Women in wedding hats give us the horrors – hats should be functional if they are to have any credibility at all. Thus straw hats look great in the sun, and wide-brimmed felt ones pulled well down over the ears look fine when it's cold. Over-sized velvet tam-o-shanters are cosy and flattering, while the truly svelte can even get away with balaclavas. Otherwise anything knitted is out, as are pastel straw jobs to match your frock. If you have to wear a hat to Ascot or a wedding, go for something impressive rather than apologetic – rise to the challenge with enthusiasm. Over forty you have the dignity and personality to wear a striking hat, whereas a pathetic one will diminish you and make you look tired. The one rule with hat-wearing is that the rest of your grooming must be perfect. Long hair usually looks better up, and the more extravagant the hat, the plainer the outfit. Make-up will need adapting too: stronger eyes and lips will balance your new head shape. Once the hat of your dreams is ensconced on your head, imagine you are a thirties movie star – they all knew how to wear hats to perfection.

GLOVES
Definitely, all the time, for any occasion. Long supple evening gloves, short leather gauntlets, driving gloves in your Porsche, all are the epitome of glamour and style.

TIGHTS
Anything dark, silky, sheer, opaque. Light only if your legs are blemish free. No patterns, especially not butterflies or such-like on the heel – they just look like you've trodden in something nasty. If flesh-coloured, they *must* be totally sheer, as nothing is more horrible than thick tan tights. Stockings are vital for steamy encounters – no man has *ever* succeeded in removing a lady's tights elegantly. (Makes you shudder to think about it, doesn't it?)

HOW TO SHOP
Designer Donna Karan told *Vogue*: 'I hate clothes – I really despise them. If I ever had to go to a store to shop I would probably have a coronary. I can't stand the pressure, I can't stand the choices, I can't stand anything about it.' So what chance do the rest of us have of shopping wisely or well?

Often the more clothes you buy, the worse you feel about yourself – the fantasy is never found, the hunger never appeased. What we crave is a simple, streamlined wardrobe, with a few items of blissful extravagance, not just more and more mediocre clothes. It's time to put your wardrobe on a diet. Throw out all the junk and resolve to feed it in future on wholesome, tasty items, with a very occasional binge on something naughty to keep the spirits high.

FEAR OF DESIGNER SHOPS
The problem with shopping in exclusive boutiques is that you need the designer outfit *before* you venture through the plate-glass door: the only way to take on the icy-indifference-bordering-on-cold-contempt of the snotty sales assistants is to act like someone so rich and famous they feel humiliated for not recognising you. If you *have* the guts to sashay in in your Marks and Sparks cardy and jeans, full marks to you. Just because the salesgirls look at you as if you keep your belongings in a pram and there's a bottle of meths clamped in your hand, it doesn't really mean they can have you banned from Bond Street. Get an attitude. Ask for the prices of things (but practise keeping your eyebrows down when they tell you) and demand to try things on. Most of all, never be tempted to buy anything just because you're in there, or because it's expensive.

In the changing room (no one is enough of a masochist to go this far in anything but her best underwear), beware of the salesperson who brings you accessories like the belt to go with the dress you're trying – she knows that with your body exposed, you'll agree to anything just to get dressed again in peace. Also when you've got your money out at the cash desk, watch out for the cunning way she points out earrings and such, thus pressurising you to make a quick (usually fatal) decision. Remember, if you've got the money to pay for a designer outfit because you've earned it, you've got the last laugh on these poor wan creatures who get paid so badly they can't afford them.

EXPANDING YOUR WARDROBE SELECTIVELY

Before buying anything, consider:

✹ *Do you have* a fundamental structure to your wardrobe? That means one basic neutral colour for your 'core' items – classic suits, jackets, skirts, coats and pants in black, grey, navy, brown (or other), to which you can add other colours. When adding new core items, always choose classics that won't date, and will work with other core items.

✹ *Are you updating* and expanding this collection each season with items that bring in the latest textures, colours, patterns, proportions and details? These are the trickiest purchases as what looks hot this summer could look dated the next. If in doubt, don't buy, or buy the Miss Selfridge version rather than a designer one.

✹ *If you want* to buy something really wild, restrict yourself to shoes, jewellery and tops that you don't mind discarding. And before buying any of these, be sure you'll wear them to death this season, because next season you won't want to.

✹ *Organise* your wardrobe by function: jackets, skirts, pants, blouses. Keep up with *Vogue* and *Elle*, and store a file of inspirational outfits. If you see something similar in a shop but it's out of season, buy it for later.

✹ *Change* cheap buttons for horn or Chanel-style gilt – adds tenners to the look of a jacket.

✹ *Buy* one or two sizes *too big*, then cut the label out when you get home – cheaper clothes are cut skimpily and they often shrink. For shirts, sweaters, T-shirts, sweat pants, look in men's departments. Add shoulderpads to droopy sweaters, take in side-seams, shorten lengths. Something that doesn't look right in the changing-room can sometimes be made perfect at home.

✹ *If you can't* afford originals, look for good designer imitations – other people can seldom tell the difference.

✹ *If you want* to give your wardrobe a nineties feel, look out for: cutaway front jackets, frock coats, parkas in velvet or taffeta, elaborate waistcoats, all-in-ones. *Colours*: bronze, gold, green, white, metallic. *Fabrics*: panne and dévoré velvet, pleated polyester, brocade, embroidery and beads.

THE DESIGNERS WHO WANT TO DRESS YOU

Azzedine Alaïa

Famous for: Provocative, short, tight, close to the body clothes – dresses for the real woman who is also very fit.

Worn by: Tina Turner, Paloma Picasso, Marie Helvin.

When to wear: When you're out looking for revenge after a broken heart.

Calvin Klein

Famous for: Elegant American sportswear, virtuously simple and pure in cut and line. His ads, by contrast, feature pictures of naked women with three or more men.

Worn by: Lauren Hutton, Anjelica Houston, Goldie Hawn.

When to wear: When feeling impossibly languorous and weary from extreme experience.

Words of wisdom: 'Women today are not there to be decorative for their husbands or boyfriends. They are not about to be decorative for anyone.' He was once quoted as saying that he only wanted women with perfect bodies to wear his clothes. Now he denies that vehemently, saying, 'A body is only a good-looking place to keep your brain warm.'

Ralph Lauren

Famous for: Clothes that echo a bygone era of restrained good taste and upper class living – in his ads characters lounge over tennis courts and polo fields with cashmere sweaters thrown over their shoulders. The very best outfits for country weekends.

Worn by: Princess Diana, Duchess of York.

When to wear: On safari, exploring the outback, country house weekends.

Giorgio Armani

Famous for: Coolly confident womanly clothes, relaxed tailoring in subtle colours, elegantly casual, perfect and easy.

Worn by: Lauren Bacall, Glenn Close, Richard Gere, Goldie Hawn, Harrison Ford.

When to wear: On TV chat shows, lunching in town, shopping in smart boutiques.

Words of wisdom: 'I hate the idea of women trying to look like children, trying to be a baby doll – it is natural to want to look younger, but adults should accept ageing, and the fashion industry should not force adults to masquerade as children.'

Donna Karan

Famous for: Streamlined, essential separates for the working woman, based around the bodysuit, wrapped skirt, cashmere blazer, strong belts and jewellery. Elegant, comfortable and very slimming.

Worn by: Barbra Streisand, Liza Minnelli, Barbara Walters, Miriam Stoppard, Patricia Hodge.

When to wear: For interviews, to work, lunching important clients.
Words of wisdom: 'I think what one tries to achieve in life is to camouflage one's hip size'; 'I'm not a model size 8 and I won't design clothes that can't be worn by a woman who is a size 12 or 14.'

Yves St Laurent

Famous for: Classic, glamorous, distinctive clothes, unbeatable jackets, dramatic evening wear. Catherine Deneuve says, 'His day clothes have a masculine quality which implies strength of character and helps a woman face a world of strangers. For evenings, when a women chooses her companions, the clothes are seductive.'
Worn by: Duchess of York, Paloma Picasso, Loulou de la Falaise.
When to wear: To fashion shows, shopping in Paris, to dinner when you want to impress.
Words of wisdom: 'I cannot pretend to do sculpture, and make a woman the ridiculous pedestal of my pretensions. To render clothing poetic, yes – but one must preserve its dignity as clothing.'

Chanel

Famous for: Uncluttered style; the collarless braid-trimmed suit, beige shoes with navy toecaps, pearls and gold chains. Wearability for the modern woman. Now designed by Karl Lagerfeld.
Worn by: Jerry Hall, Paula Yates, Selina Scott.
When to wear: Giving presentations, arriving at airports, staying at top hotels.
Words of wisdom: 'Beware of originality. In couture it leads to costume.' 'Ah no, definitely no, men were not meant to design for women.'

Romeo Gigli

Famous for: Sensual, ultra-romantic dressing. Makes dresses that are sheaths of bronze silk pleats, Byzantine metallic gold with burgundy velvet wrapped hips, chiffon dresses and cloaks embellished like altar cloths. Grace and fluidity in muted colours, deep blues, grey-greens, pale rose pink, saffron, indigo and aubergine. Fashion editors actually cry at his collections.
Worn by: Goddesses.
When to wear: When you love being a woman, to accept your Oscar, to make men fall in love with you.
Words of wisdom: 'Women can be soft yet strong; you can be a pretty woman who works, and still be feminine.'

Christian Lacroix

Famous for: Fantastical, theatrical, ornamental clothes, festooned with roses, chantilly lace, sashes, picture hats. Often completely over the top, but sometimes joyously gorgeous and colourful.
Worn by: Lucy Ferry, Madonna.
When to wear: For garden parties, Ascot, when suffering from midsummer madness.

Words of wisdom: 'I hate it when fashion it too cultured, too serious and cerebral. I prefer to have fun – life is too short to be serious.'

The Japanese look – Issey Miyake, Rei Kawakubo, Yohji Yamamoto
Famous for: Totally black clothes and asymmetric cutting – a modernist formula in opposition to Western retro dressing. Sculpted forms of pleated fabric, extraordinary designs without time, place or reference, utter simplicity and precision cutting, relying on the body for shape and movement.
Worn by: Annie Lennox, David Bowie, Tina Turner, Mick Jagger.
When to wear: To rock concerts, dinner at home, when you hate men.
Words of wisdom: 'These clothes are for modern women – women who don't need to assure their happiness by looking sexy to men by emphasising their figures, but attract them with their minds.'

Best of the British
Arabella Pollen – 'I think women understand more what other women want to wear. I do think men tend to look at women as sex objects; their response is an animal one as opposed to an intellectual one.'
Catherine Walker of Chelsea Design Company – 'I don't like separates but prefer much more structured clothes, but very simple.'
Anouska Hempel – 'Women are very complex – they come to a certain time and a certain age and they don't have to go downhill. I want them to feel secure, pleased with themselves.'
Vivienne Westwood – 'The Queen is the best-dressed woman in the world.' (She takes typically British things like tweeds, twinsets and pearls, blazers and pinstripes and twists them around – always looks eccentric but is copied by everyone.)
Also: John Galliano, Jasper Conran, Jean Muir, Nicole Farhi, Bruce Oldfield, Alistair Blair, Betty Jackson, Antony Price.

Collectibles by the legends of haute couture
Poiret – 'You must dominate women unless you want to be delivered, body and soul, to them.' He abolished the corset and invented the thin woman. Masterly cutting in loose, swathed shapes.
Balenciaga – Very strong silhouette, and great drama. Diana Vreeland said, 'His clothes were made for triumph, spectacle and drama, not for the ordinary woman.' His dresses sell at auction for around £1,000. Tina Chow has forty.
Dior – It's forty years since his New Look – tiny waists and padded hips, lampshade hats, gloves, mid-calf skirts, tulle petticoats, vast taffeta skirts with twenty-five yards of fabric, strapless ballgowns with bodices steamed into shape over horsehair hips.
Schiaparelli – Surreal, punkish clothes from the thirties: zippers on hats, safety-pins to hold sleeves, chain-fastening suits, a Dali print giant lobster on a dress. Her trademark was Shocking Pink. She said that 'women suffer from 20 per cent inferiority complexes, and 70 per cent illusions'.

FASHION FACTS AND FANTASIES

We could all be forgiven for thinking in our darker moments that the world of fashion design is dominated by out-and-out misogynists who delight in trying to make the female population look like either freaks or whores. Nobody, not even the model who pretends to enjoy wearing them on the catwalk, really *wants* to wear huge conical stitched-on breasts, masks, puffball skirts or balaclavas or even leave her breasts naked. Fashion shows have become notorious for such excesses, as designers compete in an atmosphere of hysteria to grab attention and column inches which jaded journalists willingly give them.

But recent collections seem to herald a change – designers who actually love women the way they are seem to be in the ascendant. Male and female designers do seem to be realising at last that women want clothes that *enhance* the mature female body with all its inherent curves and slopes, and are no longer willing to be distorted into flat-chested, giant-shouldered, hipless robots.

The woman over forty is really coming into her own in fashion. We can *demand* to be satisfied now that the dwindling youth market means there are more of us than of them. We are 'She Who Must Be Obeyed', and we are adamantly rejecting the little-girl image – the older woman is the new icon to replace the bimbo.

Recent collections have unveiled a new and imposing figure: tall, stately and swatched in flowing robes, she stalks down the catwalk emanating self-possession and mystique. Can it be that designers are at last regarding mature womanhood with a suitable degree of awe?

This vision of a future where just to be a woman is enough is within our grasp now, even though many of us are still so insecure about our value we feel we must go on trying to fulfil male fantasies in our daily dress. Thus we still strive to look young, thin *and* big breasted (impossible without surgical intervention, so models who haven't had implants barely exist any more), and so we go on wearing short skirts, low necklines, tight, trampy, tarty trash.

Fashion is certainly a cultural phenomenon, a barometer of the collective unconscious. It says everything about how we regard our society and the position of women in it. Sometimes it can seem like a conspiracy to make women look stupid or to keep them in their place. Their bodies are often used as a means of expressing our confusion about the female form. Much of the time fashion becomes a kind of sexual art form, fetishistic, surreal and full of veiled messages of confused desire. If we are working at a snail's pace towards a more feminist society, we can be sure that the 'woman as fetish doll' approach to fashion of the last few decades will die out, and a more elegant, dignified way of adorning the female form will appear.

Women over forty will be at the forefront of this New Age look. The catwalks will no longer be crowded with air-brained dollies, but with *real* women of all ages, stylishly swathed in the sensuous, graceful, harmonious but most of all *appropriate* clothes that we all want to be wearing today.

FOUR

What's Wrong With Your Hair?

'Getting your hair right is tremendously liberating. It opens up
whole new worlds.'

Your hair says an awful lot about you. Ask any actress – or hairdresser Stephen Way who is often asked to create hairstyles for the theatre. His comments are most revealing: 'As soon as I'm told what the character is like I know pretty quickly what kind of style I'm going to do. For instance if the brief was "create a hairdo for a downbeat, downtrodden woman, someone who'd just been left by her husband with four kids to bring up and no money," I'd do a medium length style in a drab colour, rather greasy looking and in complete disarray, with hair sticking out all over.

'For a page three Sharon or Tracy type it would be simple: blonde highlights, long at the back, short layers on top, very wide at the sides and all sort of scrunched up with lots of lacquer.

'An older woman would have to have a few grey hairs, with powder on top to make it look really dull. Perhaps permed ends too, so it was matronly and careful, but not too smart.

'If the look was a young, fashionable one then the most important thing of all would be shine. Bags of it. I'd do a sharp cut – blunt cut at the ends so it looked very thick, because this is a sign of good health. In fact the ends of the hair would have to be as strong and glossy as the roots. And it would flick about a lot whenever the woman moved.'

There you are. Not only does hair say a lot about you but it usually says it with as much subtlety as a sledgehammer. You can't ignore hair or just leave it to do its own thing, because hair is very important and as such deserves pride of place in your list of priorities. Getting your hair *right* is tremendously liberating. It opens up whole new worlds. Clothes instantly look better with a well-cut head of hair to top them off. You can actually start to *enjoy* fashion because suddenly lots of it suits you. The right haircut is better than make-up: it balances your features and face shape. The right colour flatters your eyes and skin tone.

Folklore has it that past the age of thirty 'short' is the respectable way to go – but respectable means nothing these days, it's style that counts. What you need now is stylish hair or to put it another way – hair with style.

Don't confuse stylish hair with a hairstyle though. They are two quite separate things. At forty it's tempting to rush headlong into the arms of a hairstyle thinking this is the sensible, safe, appropriate thing to do. But is it? It's easy to spot hairstyles because they usually mean you have to coax your hair to do something it doesn't really want to with lots of help from curling tongs, crimping irons, hairspray or mousse. Sometimes brute force is required and perms or razors are employed. Occasionally the soft, downy hair on the back of the neck is trimmed with clippers. Hairstyles sap individuality and foster over-dependence on hairdressers and artificial aids. Hairstyles are in constant danger of looking like hats. At their very worst they turn from hats into stiff, candyfloss helmets. Nothing is more ageing than a hairstyle that perches on top of your head like a badly chosen wig.

The thing to remember about hair is that it's sexy, sensual stuff and should move around gracefully when you do. At the very least you should be able to run your fingers through it without the end result ruining your entire day.

Technically speaking, of course, hair is dead: the trick is to make it look alive and bouncy. If you can't wash your hair and then just casually scrunch or comb it dry the chances are that you've got a hairstyle and you should seriously consider either changing your hairdresser or loosening up your own ideas a little. Always remember that hair is there to be your crowning glory, to make *you* look ravishing – not to make a statement all on its own.

Occasionally, however, the temptation to rush off to the hairdresser's for a hairstyle will be so strong that you can barely resist it. A top name hairdresser struck by inspiration from above will create a sensational new look for a famous woman that sets your pulses racing. It will probably be a soft, seductive hairstyle that frames the face prettily and leads you to believe that cocooned in a hairdo like that, you too could look like Farrah Fawcett, Joanna Lumley, Princess Di or Selina Scott. Several million other women find their pulses racing too and in the space of six months everybody looks like everybody else, and the unfortunate few – those who find this wretched hairdo really and truly *does* suit them – get stuck in a rut till the end of time. Avoid falling into this trap if you can – and get out of it fast if you're already in it.

THE PERILS OF HAIRDRESSER AVOIDANCE – OR, IF YOU WANT TO GET AHEAD GET A HAIRCUT

If you haven't set foot inside a hairdresser's for the past six months you *definitely* haven't got a hairstyle. What you have instead is hair with *no* style; this is just as bad and twice as nerve-wracking. Hair with no style has a disconcerting habit of breathing its last and going completely flat on top and droopy just when you're feeling at your most depressed and shabby. This does nothing for your face, your clothes or your self-esteem. Hair with no style is impossible to control and will stubbornly defy all your frantic attempts to perk it up. It's risky to avoid a hairdresser for more than three months at a time – this really is the absolute limit. Even the most casual of styles *must* be underpinned with a first class cut.

At forty it really is time to brace yourself for a proper haircut, even though deciding what form this should take may not be easy. Some of us will have to clear the decks of childhood trauma first. If, for instance, your mother regularly frogmarched you to the hairdresser's for a hideously shorn, convict-style haircut when you were a little girl you may well have developed a morbid fear of hairdressers and an irrational dependency on long hair now you're grown up. It's the Samson and Delilah syndrome all over again, except that this time it's reversed. You desperately need long hair in order to feel *feminine*. To have it all cut off sounds suspiciously like a sex change.

While there's no doubt that some of us actually do look much better with hair on the long side (because it suits our face shape and balances our figure), it has to be said that some of us don't. But we never get to discover this fact because we're always too scared to take the plunge. If the very thought of taking the plunge sends shivers down your spine – take it slowly instead. Book frequent appointments and let your hairdresser inch it up gradually, bit by bit.

Take heart from Mary's story. Mary finally eschewed long, brown hair in favour of a chin-length blonde bob when she was thirty-eight and found the ramifications so wholeheartedly positive that now she's cross that it took her so long.

'When I had my hair cut I finally grew up,' she explains. 'Long hair was my way of rebelling against my mother who made me wear my hair in such a short, plain way as a child that I always felt androgynous. When I got rid of the hair I shed the whole sixties, student rebellion thing and all my tatty, jumble sale clothes and denims went too.

'It didn't happen overnight. Spurred on by a new job, after five years at home, I did it in stages with my hairdresser egging me on. Having my hair bleached broke another taboo. I had such a puritanical upbringing that I spent years thinking of blonde hair as rather tarty and wicked. I was secretly envious of women with dyed hair but was too scared to do it myself.

'Once I got my hair right, my glasses had to go (I have contact lenses now) and my clothes automatically became smarter. In fact I can look rather grandly dressed on occasions. I feel altogether more poised; rather sophisticated; and confident that I look the very best I can.

'The whole experience has taught me to value my own opinions more and never to let other people put limits on my growth. All this – just from a haircut!'

The moral of this tale is: when it comes to hair it's usually better to do *something* rather than absolutely nothing at all. Even if you end up hating the cut because it's much too short or the colour is wrong, at least you will learn something useful from it. Okay, you'll learn that very short hair doesn't suit you. Big deal, you knew that all along. But while it's growing out you may well discover a new length that does.

As far as colour goes – maybe it would be a good idea to get some long-buried fantasies out of your system while you're still young enough to savour them thoroughly. It has been said that everyone should try life as a blonde or a redhead at least once. Going blonde or red has even been known to bring shy retiring types out of their shell, since there's simply no alternative but to cope with all the extra attention you receive. A word of warning here – never be tempted to have bleached streaks put in dark brown hair (it always looks dirty) or tint your hair an all over solid colour in any shade (*especially* burgundy or black). Opt for tasteful highlights or lowlights instead. They don't have to be *too* subtle.

Find a photograph of yourself fifteen years ago. If your hair today is still just the same (give or take an inch or two) then the situation is urgent. You must seek out the best hairdresser in town without delay . . .

YOU AND YOUR HAIRDRESSER

'The most important man in a woman's life is her hairdresser' – Joan Crawford

Unfortunately Joan never went on to explain how you go about finding this paragon of virtue who is worthy to become the most important man in your life because, as everyone knows, any old hairdresser just won't do. A good hairdresser, like a good man, is hard to find and when you do manage it the young, single male variety have the annoying habit of moving on (usually after your second or third appointment) to Torremolinos or California, or the Outer Hebrides or somewhere, and before you know it you're back to square one. (Married hairdressers with kids or hairdressers who own their own salons rarely do this, so they're much better bets.) You can't even pay your way to perfection. Once a brilliant hairdresser becomes rich and famous he turns overnight into a businessman and is always jetting across the Atlantic to tie up deals on his range of haircare products so he's never around for your third appointment either. The only answer is to marry the first competent hairdresser you come across (providing he's a man of course).

Of course you don't need a brilliant top name hairdresser at all, just one who understands your hair, your face (very important) and what kind of fantasy you have about how you'd like to look. Age and experience count for everything. As hairdresser Joshua Galvin points out, you don't want some good-looking young guy who spends more time gazing at himself in the mirror than he does at you. Nor do you want a scissor-happy whizz kid who's determined to send you out in the latest style no matter what, just because he wants to show off his prowess to the salon juniors. On the other hand you certainly don't want a time-warp character who's spent the last twenty years churning out shampoo and sets to the blue rinse brigade either.

All this narrows down the field quite a bit. Look for a salon owner with at least ten years' experience (that probably makes him or her thirty-plus), and who preferably trained for many years at a top name city salon (that makes him or her worldly wise, used to dealing with wealthy, fussy women of a certain age, and generally clued up).

If you can't find one of these then ask round all your friends or stop strange women with great-looking hair in the street and cross-question them. This latter advice is always given by helpful magazines who claim that the women in question are usually so flattered by the request that they tell you gladly who their hairdresser is plus anything else you may want to know.

Look before you leap

The pre-appointment consultation is another step in the right direction. This is when you go into the salon, find out who the top stylist is and then arrange to have a few words with him or her about your hair *before booking an appointment*. This gives you the opportunity to size him up. Is he really interested in what you have to say, or do his eyes keep sliding over your head to spot who's just walked in the door; does she pretend to be sympathetic to your opinions but then repeat them back completely differently? Is he too bossy, or too compliant? Could you bear to spend an hour in this person's company making stilted small talk? If you're not sure whether you've struck gold, then play safe and book up for a shampoo and blow dry or a conservative trim so you can tentatively test the water. Remember it will take several appointments anyway for a hairdresser to build up a good rapport with you and your hair.

Take in pictures

This is an excellent idea, and should never be knocked – although it often is. Okay, the odd megalomaniac *may* take offence, rip the picture up in disgust and make you feel like a worm but on the whole hairdressers are used to dealing with women who want their cut just like Goldie Hawn and don't think it's funny or strange at all. And they probably prefer them to the client who hums and haws and uses phrases like 'sort of' and 'soft' and 'not too much' and so on. A photograph gives them something real to go on and usually results in useful dialogue. Of course it needn't be a picture of a model or film star at all. It could be a picture of you, snapped at that blissful moment between cuts when your hair looked 'just right'. You'll have to be nifty with the camera though, because this phase doesn't usually last for long.

A few more tips . . .

Never let a hairdresser thin your hair, especially with a razor, unless you're absolutely convinced it's the right thing to do. Everyone in the world wants thick hair. If you've got it, you're a lucky woman and it would be crazy to let some mad fool thin it so it goes all wispy and limp.

Never just say you want a perm, *always* discuss the matter fully. There are so many different perming techniques available. Stack winding, for example, will give you a perimeter of curls around your head but leave your hair smooth at the crown. Then there's weave winding, which means that some hair is left out of every roller to give a 'messy' look (but you wouldn't want that, would you?). You may want to suggest partial perming whereby some of your hair is permed but the rest is not. Spiral winding gives even movement through one-length hair. Again pictures will help here because talk about waves and curls can get disastrously vague, and perms take months to grow out.

TOP HAIRDRESSERS SPEAK OUT

Joshua Galvin of the Daniel Galvin Salon: 'In their forties women start to do a lot more to their hair than they used to. They tint it, perm it, use hot appliances. Hair is overworked and as a result the condition suffers. It doesn't matter how much money or time you spend on your hair – if it isn't in good condition then it will look terrible. Prevention is better than cure. Treat yourself to a deep conditioning treatment every other week.

'There comes a time in a woman's life – I'd say forty-five – when long hair should either be on the floor or up and out of the way. A lot of my clients have perfected ways of putting their hair up themselves – it's usually very casually pinned, very simple, very classy.

'As far as hair goes I don't think there are any hard and fast rules as long as you wear it with style and dignity. Even a very severe style can work. Margot Fonteyn, for example, wore her hair in a tight ballet bun and she looked marvellous, it was her. And the same goes for Mary Quant, who's way past her forties, but she still looks great with a fringe and bob.

'The biggest mistake is to end up as a caricature of how you used to look. Cher and Dolly Parton spring to mind! People start talking about you behind your back, ridiculing you. Instead of saying doesn't she look marvellous for a woman in her forties and isn't she well preserved, they're laughing. The secret is to mature gracefully and with taste.'

Denise McAdam of Carey, Temple, McAdam: 'Yes, of course you can keep your hair long at forty – but within reason. If you've got a parting in the middle and it just hangs down either side of your face, dead straight, then no. But if it's styled around your face and easy to manage – no one has hours to spend on their hair these days – then that's fine. It doesn't have to be up in a bun all the time. What's the point of having long hair if you *have* to wear it up? If it only looks good when it's all coiffed up with a tiara on top, then the time has come to cut it off.

'I think the right length for long hair in your forties is just touching the shoulders. Wear it in a long bob, all one length with a fringe, or permed or coloured or layered and fluffy – it depends who's wearing it.

'Women think that men love long hair, but I don't think that's strictly true. It's just that it has a page three image. Some women think that short hair will make them look mumsy, but it needn't at all. You can wear your hair short and still look sexy but many women are terrified of losing that. Lauren Bacall and Sue Lawley have short hair and they are still very glamorous women. But there's no way I would imagine that they wake up in the morning looking that good. You have to work at it. It's not just about hair – it's clothes, jewellery, make-up too. At forty you must get everything right.'

Paul Edmonds from the Edmonds salon: 'At forty women must take into consideration that their face shape has changed. If you leave your hair too long at the sides it will frame the face and drag it down. It's better to sweep it back or up and away at the sides, which will lift the face. It shouldn't be too long either: the worst thing of all is a very girly look on an older woman. Shoulder length would be about right, but it must be well cared for – not unkempt. Layers do give extra body and volume to long hair but they're rather unfashionable at the moment.

'It's best to avoid extreme styles. If you've got very short, cropped hair and a saggy jawline or double chin, then all you'll see is the double chin. If this is your problem then what you really need is bulk and volume at ear level or higher so the emphasis is taken away from the jawline to the cheekbones and eyes.

'And very curly hair can make you look older too, because there's too much contrast. It's better to have a soft perm that only lasts for three months which you can blow dry for a sleeker, wavier look, than a very tight perm that you're stuck with for nine months. How curly your perm turns out depends largely on the size of the rollers it's set on, not the strength of the lotion used. We use bendy Molton Browners for a softer look.

'Straight one-length hair can look good, you don't *have* to have layers. I have clients in their sixties who have heavy fringes and straight hair and they look brilliant – very chic and French. But they carry the style right through – their clothes are tailored and chic too. A straight bob can be cut and styled so it's very full at the sides and brushed back to reveal the ears, or waved so there's some movement in it.

'Don't copy soap stars and *Dallas* your hair to death. Never have a hairdo that's so large it looks like a wig, or a monster that's separate from you.'

Michael Rasser of Michaeljohn: 'Throw away your rollers. Release your hair. Rollers give hair a 'set' look and too much root lift. Blow dry instead with a small brush, or scrunch dry for casual movement.

'Try to take a really objective look at yourself and decide what needs to be done. Don't get stuck in a time warp. Splash out on a good cut – a sharp, modern haircut can knock off ten years. Short is more flattering.

'One of my clients, who's in her mid-forties, has pure white hair cut in a dead straight, blunt cut bob (a bit shorter than chin length). It moves, it swings and she looks fabulous. Some women look fantastic with grey hair, but you must take care if your hair is long or it can look very witchlike.

'If you want to wear your hair up, keep it simple. Not backcombed or too elaborate. Simplicity is the key.'

Gregor at Schumi: 'You can wear long hair till you're seventy as long as you wear it with conviction and style and dress it well. French and German women cut their hair very short when they're forty but this isn't a good idea because they tend to be heavily built. Long hair can be an asset if you have a large body frame.

'Sometimes women in their forties decide to have a last fling with long hair but end up looking very dowdy if they just wear it straight with a fringe. Young girls up to the age of twenty-five can wear it like this and and look very sexy, but even *they'd* look better if they did something to it. Put some effort into it, have some layering around the face and puff it up so it looks full and bouncy and it can look tremendous at any age. Some women do suit long hair better than short – Fergie for instance. If she had asked *me* to cut her hair off, I would have said, "Think about it."

'I'm not very keen on hair that's worn "up" in a very large, full style because it can be overwhelming and make the face look heavy. Severe and sleek is best. Scooping long hair back with combs is dowdy too – if you want to wear your hair off the face it's better to achieve the same effect with the right cut. Unless hair is cut into a style it's hard to make it look good.

'The very worst style for someone with a double chin or saggy jawline would be a shingled bob that was very short at the back with a lot of hair hanging messily around the face at chin level. Instead you must expose as much of your face as you can – don't have your hair cut so it's worn over your face because this will emphasise the bad points. Reveal the forehead and nose so the eye is drawn up and away from the jawline. Don't cover up your face as you get older, let your character shine through.

'If your hair is thin and fine have a short, graduated bob that isn't longer than chin length or try a short, layered style.

'I like grey hair, but most women don't. I don't think it's grandmotherish at all and I try to talk my clients out of covering it up. I can't believe how many of them sit in front of the mirror when I've finished styling their hair and pluck out the grey hairs. I have to tell them, please do that outside the salon! I'm sure it makes the hair grow through coarse and frizzy eventually.'

EVERYTHING YOU NEED TO KNOW ABOUT LONG HAIR NOW YOU'RE FORTY

'When a woman takes her hair down, it's one of the most feminine acts there is' – *Jean Shrimpton*

❋ *Long hair is* sexy. Men with pony-tails know this too.

❋ *Long hair is* sensual and inviting to the touch.

❋ *Long hair isn't* sensual and inviting to the touch if it looks dirty or smells of cigarette smoke, which long hair often does because it's such a performance to wash and dry.

❋ *On the plus side,* long hair does take ages to look dirty because it takes grease for ever to travel even halfway down the hair shaft. For optimum conditions hairdressers recommend long hair should be washed every four or five days – no more, no less.

❋ *It's hard to look elegant* in bulky winter coats with hair draped messily around your shouders.

❋ *Long hair is the perfect accessory*, however, for glamorous evening ball-gowns. (The question is, how often do you wear glamorous evening ball-gowns?)

❋ *It's essential* to devise a nifty way of pinning long hair up.

❋ *If you don't* devise a nifty way of pinning long hair up you will have to wear a shower cap in the bath and a bathing cap in the pool and these items of headgear do nothing for self-esteem.

✸ *Brushing out* long, thick hair takes a long time (allow five minutes and *never* give up halfway through). A tangled mess at the back is the kind of blunder only the very young are forgiven.

✸ *Only the select few* will get a proper look at your neck and ears – but it's risky to skimp on hygiene.

✸ *Long full hair* can balance a tall, or plump, or heavily boned body shape. Long hair *can* make you look slimmer but this doesn't always work if you have a double chin. Avoid long hair if you're short and plump – you'll be swamped and squashed.

✸ *Is there a limit* to how long hair should be after the age of forty-five? If there is then just skimming the shoulders is probably it. Any longer drags the face down. The alternative is to wear your hair 'up' all the time, which is a daunting thought.

✸ *You can wear your hair 'up'* and enjoy all the advantages of short hair without compromising on the length or your femininity one inch.

✸ *Long hair scraped severely back* in a bun can have a curiously exciting effect on some men. It speaks of glacial control with just a hint of hidden depths. They long to unpin it and reveal the loose, wanton woman beneath. (However, this doesn't work if you go too far and look like a frumpy schoolmarm instead – you must be supercilious, elegant and well groomed.)

✸ *You may congratulate yourself* on all the hairdresser's bills you're saving but this is false economy. Long hair needs the worn-out ends trimmed off *at least* every eight to ten weeks if it's to look strong, healthy and at its very best.

✸ *Long hair costs a fortune* to highlight properly (using the tinfoil method) because there's so much of it and it takes the hairdresser hours to do. But it's worth it, because the roots only need re-touching every three months.

✸ *Think twice* before permanently tinting long hair all over – it can take years to grow out a colour you don't like.

✸ *Long hair can look dramatically glamorous* and youthful if it's thick and shiny, but hopelessly limp and dejected if it's not. Long is not the ideal way to wear fine, thin hair.

✸ *Long hair at forty* is for those who love to break the rules. It's cock-a-snooks to everyone who thinks it unseemly on women of a certain age. You love it, you're positive it still suits you – so why not?

Women who have worn their hair long (with varying degrees of success) throughout their forties and sometimes beyond: Jacqueline Bisset, Nanette Newman, Jilly Cooper, Gayle Hunnicutt, Coral Atkins, Cathy McGowan, Kate O'Mara.

EVERYTHING YOU NEED TO KNOW ABOUT SHORT HAIR NOW YOU'RE FORTY

'Short hair removes obvious feminity and replaces it with style' – *Joan Juliet Buck*

✸ *Short hair rejuvenates.* It lifts the face and quickens the step.

✸ *Short hair is chic,* efficient, organised.

✸ *Short hair can* make you look frumpy. Avoid this with a first class cut. Short hair doesn't have to mean a flat, skull cap style, or a military razor cut at the back. Short hair can be full, soft, feminine and flattering.

✸ *Short hair is* all about choice. There are a hundred different ways to wear a bob.

✸ *Short hair is easy* to care for. You can wash your hair every morning and still be at work on time.

✸ *It's a myth,* however, to think that short hair is always easy to care for. Steer clear of styles that only look good if you have to spend an arm-aching half hour moussing, gelling, tonging, Carmen-rollering or back-combing them into shape.

✸ *Short hair is* deliciously cool in summer, but chilly in winter.

✸ *Short hair provides* endless scope for elegance. Clothes look stylish and uncluttered without lots of fussy hair around neck and shoulders. Think how much easier it was for Princess Diana to carry off a simple, tailored look than it was for the Duchess of York when she had long hair.

✸ *Short hair gets greasy* faster than long because it's a much shorter trip from roots to ends. On the plus side it can be washed and dried in minutes which makes it perfect for sporty types, with the added bonus that it doesn't get in the way when you're rushing around.

✸ *Short hair demands lipstick.* All the attention goes to eyes and cheekbones so mouths get ignored, unless you put them firmly back on the map.

✹ *The shorter your hair* the more fun you can have with earrings. They can be as big, as small or as ridiculous as you like. Earrings also draw attention back to the mouth.

✹ *Short is the way to go* if your hair is fine and thin. Less length means less weight, means more oomph on top.

✹ *You'll become very friendly* with your hairdresser. Short styles need trimming every eight weeks, and they don't grow out evenly either (hair picks up speed around the crown due to good circulation here).

✹ *Short hair minimises* a large nose, so it's said, especially if there's some degree of volume at the back.

✹ *Take a tip* from Victoria Wood and Roseanne Barr and consider short and sleek if you're round faced and plump around the chin. Smooth, shiny bobs can look brilliant.

✹ *Very short,* close-cropped hair demands a small, well-shaped head, firm jawline and slender body. You have to be feeling very feisty indeed to wear your hair this way.

✹ *Everyone will see your neck,* so keep it clean and creamy smooth.

✹ *You can no longer use* your hair as a curtain to hide behind. This can be character-building.

✹ *Short hair is modern,* confident, self-assured. It's very grown-up.

Women who cut off their hair and never looked back: Julie Christie, Ali McGraw, Charlotte Rampling, Roseanne Barr, Selina Scott, Julie Walters.

GREY MATTERS

'Glad to be Grey' was something of a *cause célèbre* in the late eighties but as a full scale fashion trend failed to gain pace as fast as the pundits predicted. Much of the blame for this must rest on the shoulders of Barbara Bush who never managed to wear her white hair with the necessary glamour and pizazz and as a result set back the cause by years. There's no doubt that going very grey while your face is still young can be turned to your advantage in a most spectacular way – silver hair and blue eyes, for instance, are a stunning combination that's guaranteed to turn heads. Black hair with sharp, fresh streaks can make a positive statement too. But most of us don't go grey in a dramatic or positive way; we go grey in a drab and dowdy manner that begins with a sprinkling of off-white hairs and then limps on to salt and pepper. Top colourist Daniel Galvin believes that the Grey Movement is only for the select few: 'I have one client with thick, full, wiry grey hair and icy blue eyes and it looks wonderful. But on the whole I think grey can be be ageing – and long grey hair especially so.'

Grey hair, as I'm sure you know, isn't grey at all, it's white. It just looks grey when it mingles with your natural colour. When you are completely 100 per cent grey, you aren't grey at all, but pure snowy white. Most of us are genetically programmed to turn grey progressively at some point in our lives, although just how fast and how soon depends on our parents.

Women who tint their hair all their lives may never discover how grey they've gone. The rest of us are faced with the dilemma 'To tint or not to tint' – and more important, if so, how? It pays to think long and hard about how you're going to cope with your hair colour from now on, because one thing's for sure – the grey will keep on coming. If you do decide to tint it's going to become an integral part of your life and probably a costly and time-consuming part at that.

DANIEL GALVIN ON TINTING TECHNIQUES FOR GREY HAIR

What are the newest and best ways to deal with grey? If you were a client of one of the top colourists in the world, how would he suggest you go about it? Daniel Galvin, who has tinted the hair of just about everybody who's anybody (Twiggy, Bianca Jagger, Susan Hampshire, Lauren Bacall, Jerry Hall, Paula Abdul, Natasha Richardson, Sharon Maugham . . . the list goes on) gives us the benefit of his experience: 'The trick is not to go back to your natural colour. When you start to go grey – and this can happen at any time from the twenties onwards – nature is softening your natural hair colour, and you're starting to lose pigment from the skin too. Your natural colour is therefore going to be much too dark for you. It will drain the colour from your skin and make your eyes look weaker.

'On the other hand there must be some contrast between hair and skin. Hair is usually darker than skin so it's important not to make the hair too light either or the contrast is lost. If you go too light it will take all the character away from your face – and again drain away your natural colouring. Aim never to go more than two or three shades lighter than your natural colour.

'Think of hair colour as make-up. What you need are subtle colours that bring out your natural colouring and make your eyes look stronger. The best way to do this is to use the weakest products possible to achieve the simplest effect.'

Tinting tactics for up to ten per cent grey

'When you first go grey it's as though you've had natural lights put in your hair, it's just that they're the wrong colour and look grey or white or silver. You must take advantage of that by using very mild products – ideally semi-permanent rinses that last for four to six weeks and don't have any chemicals in them like peroxide.

'The idea is to tone down the white hair so it's one or two shades lighter than your natural colour, so you'll end up looking as though you've got soft lights in your hair.

'How to choose the right shade? This is my golden rule: think of the natural colour that your hair lightens up to on the ends when you're in the sun. That's the shade to go for.'

Tinting tactics for 25 per cent grey
'What you need here are soft lights – weaved in using tinfoil – maybe two shades lighter than your natural colour. Then apply a semi-permanent rinse to tone down any left-over grey and match the soft lights.

'The lights must be done with tints though, not bleach, so hair retains a lovely shine. Bleaching hair makes it dull.

'Tinted lights usually need retouching in twelve to fourteen weeks. At my salon we only ever retouch the roots. If you take the tint right through to the ends every time the hair ends up over-processed and a solid colour.'

Tinting tactics for 50 per cent grey
'You could carry on putting soft lights in the hair with a semi-permanent rinse on top. Or have an all-over tint one or two shades lighter than your natural colour which would bring down your white hair to one or two shades lighter than that. You still get the effect of lights in the hair. On medium brown hair for instance I might do an all-over tint taking it up to light brown, which in turn would tint the white hair to light golden brown. But yes, it would need to be retouched, in four to six weeks, there's nothing you can do about that.'

Tinting tactics for 75 per cent grey or more
'You'd need an all-over tint at least three shades lighter than your natural colour. Not a solid block of colour though – we never cover more than 90 per cent of the hair, so there would still be a flicker of grey shining through.

'The alternative is to have reverse lights. These are "lights" in a darker shade: the idea is to take hair back to how it looked, say, ten years ago.'

Ash brown hair, blue, green or grey eyes: Reverse lights in a charcoal shade that would give a fabulous silver fox effect.

Brown hair, brown eyes: Charcoal reverse lights again, so the eyes would be a strong feature once more. The combination of grey hair and brown eyes can make the skin look very pale.

Blonde or mousy hair, blue, green or grey eyes: Bleached highlights with a creamy-toned semi-permanent rinse on top so it looks as though you've got blonde highlights in your hair, not grey.

Mid-brown hair, hazel eyes: Warm golden, hazel or maybe even reddy tinted lights, with a semi-permanent on top to tone down the remaining grey.

'Do be very careful with red shades though because they can make the skin look very pink. If your complexion is sallow or pure white then red can look fine. But if you've got brown eyes, and a high colour with broken veins perhaps, then red is a definite no-no.'

Staying with grey
'If you want to stick with grey then use a shampoo that will keep it fresh and silvery, or go for an ash tone. Grey hair can easily pick up a yellowish tinge from central heating and smoky atmospheres, so you must counteract this.'

Home Tinting – dare you do it yourself? Of course – some of us are old hands already. Stick with semi-permanent rinses if you can, a couple of shades lighter – never darker – than your natural colour. A product such as Loving Care (made by Clairol) is excellent and covers 100 per cent grey, but offers a sensible, rather then sensational, selection of shades. You'll search in vain for warm red shades, for example, because it's tricky to include them in this kind of formulation. Take care with semi-permanent reds anyway – some will turn grey hair pink. Always follow the advice on the pack: if they're not suitable for use on grey hair they'll say so.

Don't get mixed up and use a permanent tint on your hair thinking it's a semi just because it's promoted as wash-in colour. If you find two bottles in the pack be aware that one is a developer, the other peroxide. A permanent tint is *permanent* and will shackle you to a slight regrowth problem until it grows out. And the more regularly you use a permanent tint, the more obvious this regrowth will be.

Don't mess with home highlighting kits unless you're a compulsive risk-taker or love wearing hats. Of course some women do highlight their hair successfully at home, usually with help from a friend. They must do or manufacturers wouldn't keep on making the kits. But experiments like this can go wrong in a spectacular way. The best-looking highlights are those woven in by your hairdresser using tinfoil. Expertly done up, regrowth is so subtle it's hardly any problem at all.

SHINY, HEALTHY HAIR – YOUR FOUR STEP CAMPAIGN
Shiny hair is seen as a sign of good health but this is nonsense really because hair is dead matter. It's much more likely to be a sign of someone who has looked after her hair with scrupulous care and tireless attention to detail. The bad news is that from now on you will have your work cut out to achieve shiny hair because as we get older so the odds slowly stack against us. Each individual hair shaft gets progressively thinner from the age of twenty onwards and due to structural changes within the hair shaft, slightly stiffer too. There's also a slow but steady decline in the production of hair's natural conditioner, sebum. You don't need gallons of sebum, though, to have shiny hair. Much more important is an undamaged, sleek, flat cuticle. The cuticle protects the hair shaft and is made up of transparent, overlapping scales: think of roof tiles and you'll get the idea. Anything that ruffles up, tears or damages the cuticle results in dull, lacklustre hair, and also allows moisture

to escape from the hair shaft which makes hair rather brittle too. Well-known cuticle rufflers include bleach (number one villain), permanent tints, perms, heated appliances of every description and general rough handling with brushes, towels, hair accessories and so on. In other words, just about everything you're likely to do to your hair except condition it or comb it gently through will go some way to wrecking its shine potential. Your only hope is to adopt minimum damage tactics in every area of your haircare strategy. Here's how:

Step One: Attention to lifestyle Of course it goes without saying that a well-balanced diet is essential to healthy hair growth but we'll say it anyway. Poor diet can be reflected in hair quality to quite an amazing degree: dandruff, dry hair and even hair loss (especially if you're anaemic, or short on nutrients due to crash or cranky dieting) can result.

What else can help in your quest for healthy, shiny hair? Some trichologists stress the importance of the B vitamins, aerobic exercise to stimulate circulation to the scalp and relaxation techniques to lower stress. Some are convinced stress can be a key factor in both dandruff and hair loss, although there's little medical evidence available at the moment to support these ideas. Either way don't expect to see the results of a new health regime by next week. Hair grows fast by the body's standards – half an inch a month – but that's a snail's pace for anyone impatiently waiting to see an improvement in condition.

Step Two: Scalp work-out Anything that encourages the blood supply to the scalp may be helpful, so exercise again fits in here, particularly if it's the kind that involves a lot of bending over or standing on your head! The less energetic or more stiff-jointed amongst us will have to rely on a daily (if possible) scalp massage instead (which is probably a pretty good way to tone up flabby upper arms as well). Take your time over it and you will reap some pleasurable relaxation benefits too.

Begin at the nape of your neck, and use the pads of your fingertips; keep your nails well clear and don't use your entire hand. Gently rotate your scalp (not hair) with circular movements, travelling towards the crown of your head. Do this in a slow gentle fashion and it will take a minute or even two. Now exert a little more pressure as you move towards your hairline. At the same time use your thumbs to move over your ears towards the temples. Make small circles all along your hairline, lifting your hair out of the way as you go. Relax, sit back and enjoy the slightly tingly sensation you will feel in your scalp. Do it all over again if you're in the mood.

Step Three: Routine maintenance Get your day-to-day shampooing and conditioning routine down to a fine art. The buzzword at the moment is build-up. Build-up is the prime reason why the shampoo that has worked like magic on your hair for the past couple of weeks produces a mediocre, floppy headful of hair on your fifth or sixth attempt. Many shampoos and conditioners are loaded with additives these days, and they build up on the hair shaft with regular use leaving a dull film on the hair. Switching products is usually all you need to do, but if you want to be really fashionable you'll look for a plain unadorned shampoo (such as that made by Neutrogena) and give your hair a proper spring-clean.

If you wash your hair a lot, counteract the drying effects by diluting the shampoo with water. If you do this you may be able to get away with using even less than the regulation 'blob as big as a ten pence piece'. The more you wash your hair the more you are likely to need just one wash rather than two. Scrupulous rinsing is a must. Any shampoo left behind on the hair is guaranteed to make it look dull – and that goes for cream rinse conditioners too. Cream rinse conditioners are a vital adjunct to the shampooing ritual; they ensure that the cuticle is left lying flat and pave the way for a safe, painless comb-through at the end. Finish with a cider vinegar rinse (one part vinegar, seven parts water) if you want to be really certain that your hair is tickety-boo clean (it's an old-fashioned shine restorer too). Blot your hair gently with a towel, don't rub vigorously, and let it dry naturally if possible. If it isn't possible then protect hair with a blow dry lotion when blow drying, keep the nozzle well away from your head and point it down the hair shaft, not up, which will ruffle the cuticle. Best of all, dry with a diffuser attachment or infra-red dryer which produce a much gentler form of heat.

Step Four: Conditioning treats Find the time to pamper your hair with a deep conditioning treatment as often as possible (once a week if you think it needs it). There are two ways to go about this: either give yourself a pre-shampoo oil treatment, or a post-shampoo conditioning treatment. For the oil treatment use an ordinary vegetable oil like safflower or sunflower, or splurge on a top class oil like jojoba (stocked by the Body Shop). Apply with a pastry brush and then wrap your hair in hot damp towels or hide it under a shower cap and then wrap it in hot damp towels. Leave it luxuriating in the oil for as long as possible and then shampoo your hair twice, and finish with a cream rinse.

Alternatively take your pick from the ever expanding range of deep conditioners to be found on the market these days. Protein conditioners are particularly useful if your hair has been chemically tampered with by permanent tints, bleach or perms, as they go some way to filling in any damaged, holey bits in the hair shaft. It's only temporary help though. You don't have to stick to the recommended treatment time – put on a shower cap and have a bath and spin it out for as long as you can.

LOSING YOUR HAIR

Hair loss is a terrifying thing, all the more so because few of us know much about it. Small wonder, for the list of possible causes is alarmingly long. Your hair fall may be patchy, leaving you with smooth, round, isolated bald spots, or it may be diffuse, in which case your hair may begin to feel thinner (sometimes finer) all over. Some women notice that they are beginning to recede at the temples and thin at the crown like a man. Others go totally bald. It has been estimated that over 1.6 million women in the UK suffer from hair loss at some point in their lives.

Over the last few years we have started to hear a lot about hair loss. Male pattern baldness (which affects many women too) hit the headlines with the discovery that a blood pressure drug called minoxodil (trade name Regaine) could stimulate hair growth. The knock-on effect was an upsurge of interest in the problem in medical circles. Less dramatically, but no less welcome for that, TV journalist Elizabeth Steel, who suffered almost total baldness as a result of alopecia areata, wrote a book called *Coping with Sudden Hair Loss* (Thorsons). She aired her own experiences, related numerous case histories, and offered reassurance and detailed information on medical treatments available. In short she opened up the subject and brought hope and comfort to thousands.

WHAT CAUSES HAIR LOSS

At its most innocuous hair fall can be a seasonal thing. At the Scalp and Hair Hospital (run by the Institute of Trichologists) consultant John Firmage says that many patients turn up complaining of increased hair fall in spring and autumn. It's usually just a passing phase, but no less worrying for that. He believes that over-exposure to sun and sea can aggravate the problem.

It's considered perfectly normal to lose anything from 20 to 100 hairs every day. This sounds a lot but isn't when you consider there are 90,000 to 140,000 hairs on the average person's head and they're all in varying stages of growth and rest. At any one time you can probably reckon that 90 per cent of your hair will be in the growing phase, while 10 per cent will be resting; new hairs growing through usually push the resting hairs out.

HAIR FALL AND PREGNANCY

It has been estimated that up to 45 per cent of women suffer considerable hair loss after the birth of a baby, although hair does not usually start to fall until three months later. The reason for this is hormonal.

When a woman is pregnant the levels of the hormone progesterone are unusually high and this has the effect of pushing hair into the resting phase prematurely. After pregnancy, when hormone levels re-balance, new hair begins to grow and eventually pushes the resting hairs out. When hair begins to fall it's usually a good sign that new growth is on the way. However, the fall can last for up to six months and many women find their hair never regains its former luxuriant thickness. All you can do is eat a well-balanced diet to ensure that hair has all it needs for healthy growth and treat it with care.

For the same reasons, coming off the contraceptive pill may cause temporary hair fall too.

COMMON THINNING

According to Dr David Fenton of the Dowling Hair Unit of St John's Dermatology Centre at St Thomas's Hospital in London, most women experience common thinning to some degree: 'It's the same sort of thing that affects men, but women don't get it earlier because they're protected by the high levels of oestrogen in their bodies. When these levels start to fall around the time of the menopause the male hormones (androgens), which women have in their bodies too, begin to play a more dominant role.'

It's the action of the male hormones on the hair follicles that results in shorter, finer, wispier hair growth than normal, sometimes accompanied by a thinning of hair on top of the head and a receding of growth around the hairline at the front. Some people have hair follicles that are sensitive to androgens and others don't. Common thinning is usually an inherited condition. Some women, like men, are genetically programmed to lose their hair in this way, but nowadays treatment may be offered. 'Hormone Replacement Therapy can help,' says Dr Fenton. 'Sometimes anti-androgens combined with oestrogens taken by mouth are prescribed for younger women. Anti-androgrens, however, may halt the progression of hair fall, but they seem to have very little effect on the growth of new hair.

'Another way to use anti-androgens is to apply them topically, directly to the scalp in lotion form, but so far results have been disappointing.

'Minoxodil is more commonly used. It comes in lotion form in an alcohol base in concentrations ranging from 2 to 5 per cent, and is applied directly on to the scalp twice a day. This can have several effects. It can slow down thinning or halt it completely. It can thicken the hair that you already have so each individual hair shaft grows through thicker, or it can encourage new hair to grow. The younger you are, the sooner you seek treatment, and the smaller the area that has to be treated, the better the results are likely to be. It's a very slow improvement, however, not a dramatic one.

'Minoxodil is a useful treatment, but in our research we find that using a concentration higher than 2 per cent gives better results. It is safe provided you use it under medical supervision in the right quantities, so very little is absorbed into the body. But unfortunately as soon as treatment stops the thinning returns.

'The other way to approach the problem, if it's severe, is with hair transplants. I've seen some marvellous results. However, I must stress very strongly how important it is to find a skilled surgeon. The successes I've seen have been on patients who have travelled abroad to highly experienced surgeons who employ very sophisticated methods. They transplant single hair follicles so it's a very lengthy procedure. And, of course, extremely expensive too.'

ALOPECIA AREATA

Alopecia areata means patchy baldness, although some people go on to lose all their hair (alopecia totalis), while others lose all their body hair too (alopecia universalis). Around 2 per cent of the population suffer from this problem at some stage in their lives. The good news is that in most cases the hair does grow back – eventually.

A lot of people have alopecia areata and don't even know they've got it, according to one dermatologist: 'A small patch on the back of the head, for instance, may go unnoticed. I've had it myself – tiny bald spots on the beard. Current evidence suggests that it's an auto-immune disease, although this may be coupled with an inherited predisposition to it.

'There's no real evidence that it's caused by nerves. Ask someone if they've suffered stress within the last three to six months and most will say that they have, although when it follows something like a bad car accident one can't help feeling that it's more than coincidence.'

There are a wide variety of treatments available. A doctor or dermatologist may prescribe minoxodil, steroid creams, cortisone injections into the scalp, Psoralen and Ultra Violet Therapy (PUVA) . . . all may have varying degrees of success in stimulating regrowth. See your GP first and if he is unwilling to offer first line treatment, ask for a note to see a dermatologist. As Elizabeth Steel says, 'You may have to batter down doors to find experts who will help.'

OTHER POSSIBLE CAUSES OF HAIR LOSS

If you are anaemic this can cause excessive hair fall. Consult your doctor: a course of iron tablets may be all that's needed to sort the problem out.

An underactive thyroid also leads to increased hair fall and this may be one of the first symptoms you notice. Many women suffer thyroid dysfunction after childbirth which, coupled with post-pregnancy hair fall, sometimes confuses the issue.

High fevers or a local skin problem with the scalp are two more possible causes of hair loss. In fact persistent hair fall can be a symptom of such a wide variety of underlying health problems that it's always wise to consult a doctor if you're worried.

MAKE PEACE WITH YOUR HAIR

It really doesn't matter if your hair is long or short, thick or thin, grey or tinted. What does matter desperately is that it is expertly and regularly cut, lovingly and constantly conditioned. Hang-ups about your hair that keep you out of the hairdressers for months or even years at a time must be conquered once and for all. Don't let the odd disaster deter you in your quest for the haircut that has your name well and truly stamped on it. This is unlikely to be a style that is extreme or quirky in any shape or form. Don't waste time experimenting with those tight frizzy perms so popular amongst footballers in the seventies for instance. Contrived, messy styles that need to be stiff with mousse and require constant tweaking will bring you no joy either. Celebrity hairdos look great for five minutes but have a very short shelf life. Anything reminiscent of Farrah Fawcett in her heyday should be given a wide berth too.

Don't be afraid to take the odd risk. Don't become hidebound by convention. Find a hairdresser you can trust and listen to him. Fabulous hair can be yours as long as you're prepared to keep on trying.

FIVE

Refresher Course For Skin

'A face without lines is like a book without words'
Elizabeth Arden

'Please don't re-touch my wrinkles, it took me so long to earn them'
– actress *Anna Magnani* speaking to a photographer.

Forget grey hairs, they mean nothing in the grand scheme of things. It's wrinkles that deal the hardest blow of all. They are nothing less than our first intimations of mortality. Compared to this every other aspect of growing older is a doddle. We can, after all, do much to protect our health (and improve our figures) with sound nutrition, exercise and check-ups; we can tint our hair and cover the grey; we can dress with elegance and make up with expertise. But skin has a mind of its own. It's not as biddable as the rest – what can we do about skin except put on a brave face and pray?

Actually quite a lot. As far as our skin goes we are both the luckiest and unluckiest of women. Unlucky because when we were young the cult of sun worship hit its peak and we were affluent enough to indulge ourselves with holidays abroad. Unlucky because getting a tan has become a habit that some of us are surprisingly unwilling to break (how many times do we have to be told that a tan now means wrinkles later?)

But we're lucky too. Thanks to scientific research we now know how to avoid ageing skin prematurely (it's *never* too late to take preventive measures) and how to look after it in the simplest, most effective way. Many dermatologists, once chary of the beauty business, are beginning to join in the skincare debate. As a result we are much better equipped to sort the facts from the hype and the hype from the plain untruths. The message is clear – state of the art skincare is easy, relatively cheap and available to us all. There's much to do, and much to look forward to . . .

WHAT ON EARTH HAS HAPPENED TO YOUR SKIN?

Coco Chanel once said that when we're fifty we get the face we deserve, but that's only partly true. There's no doubt that lifestyle does play a big part: sun, smoking, crash diets, stress, they can all wreak havoc with skin and are well-known fast-agers. But we also get the skin and the face (and all faces age differently – it's not *just* about skin) that we've inherited from our parents.

When doctors talk about skin they like to talk about intrinsic and extrinsic ageing. Extrinsic ageing is the ageing we inflict on ourselves, while intrinsic ageing just happens – whether we like it or not. Let's consider first what's likely to happen to your skin however calm, reclusive and clean living you've been:

❋ *Count yourself lucky* if your ancestors have bestowed upon you high, prominent cheekbones and a strong jawline, because these will support your skin like scaffolding over the years and help to offset the effects of sagging. (Where, for instance, would Joan Collins be without those fabulous cheekbones?) Plastic surgeons will love you too. It's much easier for them to redrape skin over a strong bone structure. Don't expect to get off scot-free though: everyone's bones begin to shrink from the age of thirty onwards.

❋ *Take a look* at a picture of yourself when you were sixteen and you'll be struck by how *fat* your face looked then. When we're young our skin is generously padded out with plenty of underlying fat, which acts as a nice bouncy cushion for skin to sit on. The good thing about having a plump face is that the extra padding irons out wrinkles. However, we all experience some shrinkage of this fat layer over the years.

※ *In our forties* both the top layer of skin (the epidermis) and the layer underneath (the dermis) begin to thin out too. The dermis is made up largely of an elastic tissue called collagen (you read about it all the time on jars of anti-wrinkle cream). Collagen has been likened to many things in its time, but a mattress probably fits the bill best. In an ideal world fibres of collagen lie in neat parallel bundles interwoven with strands of elastin (elastic tissue), to give skin its tensile strength, its youthful spring and bounce. Hormones play a large part in how much collagen the body produces; supplies begin to falter when oestrogen levels drop as a result of the menopause.

※ *At least some of our facial droopiness* can be blamed on gravity, which has been trying to drag our face in a depressingly downward direction ever since we were born. With less support from underlying tissues, some people notice that the lower part of their cheeks begins to drop, creating a jowly effect around the jawline. The nose seems to get longer too, and on older people there's a marked elongation of the earlobes.

※ *Smiling, laughing, frowning, squinting* – the more you move your face around in daily life, the more expression lines you're likely to have. Wear and tear on underlying collagen eventually leads to permanent creases. The furrowed brow refuses to smooth out even when you're relaxed and there are laughter lines around your mouth.

※ *Your skin tone* is lighter because you don't produce as much melanin as you used to. Aha! That explains why it's so difficult to get a tan these days! The rosy glow of youth has gone and it takes a great deal to make you blush. Circulation to skin is less efficient, so there's less blood to bring oxygen and nourishment for cell renewal and repair to carry away waste products.

※ *Subtle changes* are taking place too. The texture of your skin is likely to feel rougher and look dull. Your skin is not as well lubricated as it used to be because the sebaceous glands in the dermis (they pipe oil straight on to the skin's surface) have begun to shrink and reduce their flow. This is great news for acne sufferers, but not so hot for those with dry skin. Dead cells hang around on the surface of skin for a lot longer than they used to. And new cells are produced at a much slower rate.

THE BEST ANTI-WRINKLE CREAM ON THE MARKET

The best anti-wrinkle cream on the market is, of course, a total sun block, which is not, we suspect, the answer you were hoping to hear. (There is another excellent anti-wrinkle cream on the market too, but that merely rectifies the wrinkles you acquire by not wearing the best one.) It must be admitted that sun blocks are not the most exciting of products. There's no immediate pay-off for a start, certainly no promise of 'firmer skin in three weeks', and to cap it all, not even a tan. But consider this: *99 per cent of wrinkles are caused by sun damage: 1 per cent are the result of natural ageing.*

'Almost all the skin changes that people really don't like – wrinkling, roughness, sagging, bumps, irregular pigmentation, sallow skin tone – are attributable to sun damage, not age,' says Professor Barbara Gilchrest of the Boston University School of Medicine. 'As recently as the sixties,' she says, 'it was believed that all the changes people saw and experienced with their skin were due to intrinsic ageing, just the process of getting older. Now we know that much of the problem is directly due to sun exposure – we call it photoageing.

'Sun exposure is also very closely related to skin cancer. The overwhelming majority of skin cancers occur in the maximally exposed areas of the body.

'We have already made substantial progress in the area of prevention. In every corner drug store there are compounds which will block out the damaging rays of the sun.'

The sneaky thing about sun damage is that it creeps up on you stealthily, like a stranger in the night. You think you've got away with it, but no one does. Five, ten, fifteen years later your face begins to reveal your suntanning habits for all the world to see. The damage logs up year by year and begins in childhood. Professor Albert Kligman, world-renowned dermatologist of the University of Pennsylvania, reckons he has never examined a fifteen-year-old white woman with 'normal' skin. 'Every person aged fifteen who has been able to go on vacation and go to the beach and sunbathe does not have normal skin. It is already structurally spoilt.'

We have all been aged to some extent by the sun. There's no avoiding day-to-day exposure to ultraviolet light, unless you become a Buddhist monk and stay indoors all your life. Dr Kligman found one once and reported that at ninety-six years old his skin was as smooth as a 'baby's bottom', and as everyone knows you can't get much smoother than that.

GOOD REASONS TO START USING A SUN BLOCK NOW

The sensation of sun beating down on bare skin is very heaven, but the effects can be long term and hellish. We pay the price of a tan with some-times devastating damage to our skin. Some of us have discovered that already. Every time you are tempted to turn an unprotected face skywards in expectation of a golden glow, stop for a moment and think hard about what the consequences might be:

☀ **Thick, leathery skin.** The skin responds to UV radiation by valiantly thickening up the dead cell layer in order to protect itself. Following years of chronic exposure this becomes a permanent fixture.

❋ *Increased risk of skin cancer.* Damage to the DNA of epidermal cells by ultraviolet radiation can result in pre-malignant changes which will one day lead to skin cancer. Sunburn in childhood doubles the risk of skin cancer in adult life.

❋ *Sagging skin and wrinkles.* The elastin fibres which help to keep skin supple first thicken and then over the years disappear. Collagen begins to harden and distintegrate. The epidermis collapses inwards forming wrinkles, creases and folds.

❋ *Broken blood vessels.* Blood vessels, which are being produced by the skin all the time, dwindle in number. There are far fewer channels to bring nourishment to the skin. Some become permanently dilated due to lessening support from surrounding collagen or over-stretching of the vessel walls.

❋ *Sallow skin and age spots.* Skin produces the brown pigment melanin as its second line of defence against UV radiation. Melanin is a very good natural sunscreen if your skin is capable of producing enough. Fair skins aren't. But the skin does try. In fact it goes a little crazy and deposits clumps of brown pigment in the basal layer of the epidermis, which never quite make it to the top. As our skin tone lightens over the years they become more noticeable.

It's impossible to acquire a tan without doing some damage to the skin in the process, however slowly and carefully you go about it. A tan is the skin's response to attack, not an insurance policy against it. Wearing a sunscreen will minimise the harm, not preclude it. To do that you must use a sun block – *and stay pale.* Tan your body a little if you want to, but at least, please, protect your face.

Two more good reasons to be extra fussy about sunbathing from now on: you've less chance of getting as tanned as you did in your youth because melanin production has slowed down. The longer you spend trying, the more damage you'll log up. Added to this the thinning of the ozone layer has coincided with an increase in skin cancers. The Royal College of Physicians recommend we use a sunscreen with a Sun Protection Factor of at least 6 all through our holidays in the sun.

You don't have to spend a fortune on sunscreens. There are only so many sunscreen ingredients that pass muster and you'll find them in the poshest and the most humble brands. Don't buy a sunscreen unless it offers protection from UVB *and* UVA rays. UVB rays are the short wave rays that burn skin and stimulate a tan, but long wave UVA rays, although they don't burn and only tan skin at a snail's pace, are the *slow insidious agers of skin.* Their rays penetrate right to the heart of the matter – the dermis – and they're the reason why we all have some degree of sun damage to the skin whether we sunbathe or not. But, and it's a big but at the moment, sunscreens can't claim to give you measured protection from UVA (the SPF number only applies to UVB) because testing is tricky. Doctors are working hard right now to rectify the situation. You can help yourself here by buying sunscreens with particles of titanium dioxide or zinc oxide in them because these provide a physical barrier (not total) against all forms of UV light.

On the beach, or out in the country on sunny summer days, apply your sunscreen generously. When testing in the labs in Britain the men in white coats use 1.3 milligrammes of sunscreen per square centimetre of skin. The American companies use 2 milligrammes per square centimetre of skin (one reason why their SPFs are always higher). Most people use half that amount. And put it on half an hour before you go out in the sun – sunscreens need that time to form a bond with the skin. Go on re-applying every few hours.

FAKE IT

Just because you don't want to tan your face any more doesn't mean you can't look as though you have. Smart women use a fake tan – sparingly. Fake tan has it over make-up for summer days because it's easy to keep applying sunblock on top, whereas smearing sunblock on top of make-up just isn't practical. Luckily there are now products available designed for the face which don't contain so much of the staining chemical involved (Dihydroxyacetone or DHA) so the effects are subtle and can be built up slowly. Everyone reacts to DHA slightly differently; it depends on the balance of amino-acids in the top layer of your skin. Prepare skin by exfoliating and moisturising lavishly, especially when you're using the product on the body. Dark patches usually form where the skin is driest. Knees, elbows, heels can be dead giveaways.

ACTION PLAN FOR SKIN

You probably have your skincare routine down to a fine art by now. Cleanse, tone/wash, moisturise is still your best bet as a daily maintenance plan. The only difference is that from now on you must follow it more scrupulously and attentively than ever before.

Does it need a little fine-tuning? Probably. Skin changes its behaviour from month to month, season to season, year to year. You may have become rather fond of thinking of yourself as an oily or normal skin type when that classification no longer holds true. It may be time for a change of products along with a few simple additions to your daily or weekly routine.

CLEANSING

Skin looks better when it's clean. Dead skin cells, wax-based make-up, atmospheric pollution, good old-fashioned dust and dirt, with the addition of natural skin secretions must all be cleaned off as thoroughly as possible every night or skin soon responds by looking dingy and grey. Wearing your make-up to bed just means you're presented with twice as much work in the morning and skin gets too much stimulation in one go: cleansing, toning, moisturising and then more make-up slapped on top before it's had time to recover its equilibrium, re-balance its protective acid mantle (a mixture of oils, sebum and sweat) or slough off dead skin cells.

Most make-up isn't water-soluble so oil-based cleansing creams and lotions are a must. Whether they're heavy and creamy or light and milky is a matter of personal choice, the only proviso being that you give your skin at least two goes with them.

You'll need to follow cleansing with skin toner. Its function is to remove the oily residue left behind by the cleanser (not to close pores which, incidentally, nothing on this earth can do). If you prefer to wash with soap and water instead then that's fine, but make it the mildest you can find and if you live in a hard water area choose a detergent bar instead. Soap plus hard water combines to form minute and sometimes irritating mineral deposits which can easily be left behind if rinsing isn't super-thorough. (Why else do you think the prestigious Erno Laszlo regime demands sixty splashes a day to rinse off their status-symbol Black Mud Soap?)

EXFOLIATION

The women who need to exfoliate most are usually the last to take it on board. That's us, the fortysomethings, and we'll go on needing to do it more and more as the years go by.

The rationale behind this directive is a sound one: exfoliation makes skin look, and even temporarily behave, as though it were a few years younger. The premise is simple: skin cells are manufactured (by a process of cell division) in the basal cell layer of the epidermis and then slowly migrate to the surface of the skin, the bit we see, treat and touch every day. By the time they reach the top they are flattened, packed tightly together and quite dead. Eventually, by fair means or foul, they are sloughed off in a cloud of microscopic dust. (Did you know that 60 per cent of the dust in the vacuum cleaner is dead skin cells?) In a young person the whole cycle from start to finish takes twenty-eight to thirty days. In an older skin it can take forty-five days or more. As a result the cells sitting on top of our skin are likely to be more tired out and more damaged than those of our younger sisters. And they love to clump together in tiny, uneven lumps and then refuse to budge. If we can remove this unnecessary debris either mechanically or chemically, then fresher, younger, more transparent skin will be revealed. Moisturising creams can do their job more efficiently on top of smooth, debris-free skin, and sluggish cell production is given a temporary shot in the arm.

One of the best and gentlest ways to exfoliate skin is with a complexion brush and soap and water (or face wash or complexion bar). The Buf-Puf, a polyester fibre sponge, comes highly recommended too. Slide it over the skin – don't rub vigorously though, let its rough texture do the job for you. Scrub creams are great too, but can work out an expensive addition to your cleansing routine: choose ones that have synthetic rounded granules rather than those based on natural ingredients which can be a bit scratchy. Some toner-type products offer an exfoliation service too. Usually alcohol-based, they work chemically by breaking down the cohesive bonds between dead skin cells so they can easily be wiped away. Look at the cotton wool after you've finished using one and prepare to be shocked by its dirty grey colour.

FACE MASKS

These perform much the same job as exfoliators but with a few more airs and graces so they're not suitable for everyday use. They may contain ingredients such as menthol, which dilates blood vessels, or clay which absorbs dirt and grease.

The best face packs to use now could well be the fruity ones that you make up yourself. This is because some fruits and vegetables (notably citrus fruits and apples) contain an acid called AHA (Alpha Hydroxy Acid) which is very clever at promoting the shedding of dead skin cells. As a result one American dermatologist found that by treating patients with very dry skin with a solution of AHA, many of their wrinkles, age spots and surface acne scars seemed to disappear too. I'm not suggesting that you'd get such miraculous results with a fruit mask but you will be left, at the very least, with clean, soft skin. Make up a fruit-based mask by pulverising an apple, orange or lemon and then mixing with natural yoghurt or fine oatmeal. Or simply wipe over your skin with a slice of lemon, orange or tomato.

MOISTURISE

Wearing a moisturiser won't make a jot of difference to how fast your skin shows its age (unless it contains a jolly good sunscreen) but it will make more than a jot of difference to how your skin looks and feels.

Skin needs moisture supplied from within to keep surface cells plump and smooth. Skin looks marginally younger when it's well moisturised and it takes on a healthier colour too.

A moisturiser's most important job is to keep water in the skin, not to add to it. Think of it as inefficient cling film, trying its hardest to seal moisture in the skin with a layer of fine oils. Dermatologists like Albert Kligman sing the praises of Vaseline. Well, it probably is the nearest to cling film you can get, but unsurprisingly there are few takers on this one. The next best thing would be a product that contains some petrolatum – Nivea for instance.

Because 'occlusion' is the name of the game it makes sense to opt for slightly heavier creams; your skin is likely to be drier now and anyway fine lines look better when they're nicely plumped up. Light, water-in-oil formulations are tempting because they're featherlight on the skin, but the water content evaporates in minutes (sometimes taking some of your skin's own moisture with it) leaving a finer, less effective layer of oil behind. Someimes skin actually feels drier a little while after use.

Become your own consumer watchdog: test moisturisers before buying on the back of your hand. If they disappear quickly and leave your skin feeling cool, they're probably too light for the job. Some foam up horribly when you're smoothing them in. This is because moisturisers are basically made from oils and water and refined detergents ('emulsifying agents' sounds better, doesn't it?) – this last element is vital or the oil and water won't mix. However, too much foaming, which takes ages to get rid of, suggests a crude formulation.

Added ingredients bump up the price. Most moisturisers these days contain some humectants, because they're good at retaining water and keeping it in the skin. Urea, for instance (found naturally in sweat), is a popular one. Phosopholids and lactic acid are good humectants too. Some humectants are so good that they draw moisture from the atmosphere into the skin. Glycerin, for instance, works well in humid climates (where paradoxically your moisturising needs would be less anyway) but is best avoided when the atmosphere is dry, because then it tends to draw moisture up from the skin itself to satisfy its thirst.

Ingredients that can make moisturisers very pricey indeed are Hyaluronic acid, occurring naturally in the dermis and a world class humectant (found in some of the swankiest creams); cerebrosides (lipids similar to those found in cell membranes); and ceramides (lipids again but this time mimicking the inter-cellular cement that binds dead cells together). The best added ingredient of all? Sunscreen, of course.

Just as important as moisturising is control of the environment you spend most time in, especially in winter. Low humidity levels rob skin of moisture and central heating and air conditioning are lethal. A humidifier will keep the atmosphere perfectly balanced; alternatively place bowls of water on radiators, desks and tables and surround yourself with plants.

DO YOU NEED AN ANTI-AGEING CREAM?

This is a big decision because the money involved can reach dizzying heights. The trouble with most 'anti-ageing' creams is that you need more than an A level in Biology to grasp what they claim to do in the first place (often, it turns out, surprisingly little) and then you need to be at least a dermatologist to understand if they've a hope in hell of actually achieving it. In the end you're either a believer or you're not. Amongst those who are not you will find many dermatologists. The most eminent of these are recruited from time to time by one national newspaper or another to cast their beady eyes over a selection of high-tech creams and then pass judgement. They invariably pooh-pooh all the jargon and high-flown claims, but concede that the products probably *are* jolly good moisturisers. (Some however are not even that, requiring you to wear a moisturiser on top.) Undeterred, the cosmetic companies carry on spending millions of pounds between them on ever more sophisticated technology to help them in their tireless research: developing, refining and testing new ingredients and formulations. You can't deny they're trying, and some of them very hard at that. A spokeswoman for Lancôme summed up their position thus: 'Anti-ageing is probably a marketing term that people overuse, but no one can argue with the fact that sun filters and top quality, expensive ingredients like macademia oil do nourish dehydrated skin and protect it from sun damage, so in that way they are age preventative. There's no doubt that if you use a cream like Niosôme your skin will be in better condition than if you didn't. Whenever magazines run two or three week consumer trials our products usually come out very well.'

There's no doubt too that paying a fortune for a jar of skin cream can have important spin-off benefits. You're much more likely to *use* it in a regular and serious way if you've paid plenty. However, it's as well to be aware of two points:

Fact One Any product that contains sun filters is perfectly justified in claiming that it's anti-ageing. I know of at least one night cream that incorporates sun filters in its formula.

Fact Two All wrinkles originate in the dermis. Most companies don't claim that their ingredients can reach that far. And if they do then some dermatologists argue that to expect them to do anything useful once they get there is hoping for the impossible. If they *were* actually capable of altering the physiology of living cells they would cease to be cosmetics and become drugs.

In the late eighties claims for anti-ageing products reached fever pitch, and the American Food and Drug Administration stepped in. They demanded that companies drop their claims of physiological effects on the body or their cosmetics would be seized or reclassified as drugs. (It costs huge sums of money to test new drugs.) Most dropped their claims, and American beauty writers started talking about a new age of 'modesty' that was abroad in the land. Our own Department of Trade and Industry has also written to the Cosmetic, Toiletry and Perfumery Association asking its members not to make claims that they can't fully substantiate.

As a result the temperature has cooled. At Lancôme, for instance, they are concentrating their efforts on ways to provide protection from ultraviolet light in creams for everyday use, and new and better ways to hydrate the skin. It sounds like good sense. A good moisturiser and a sun block are still the best anyone can buy over the counter at the moment to protect, enhance and cherish the skin.

COUNTER STRATEGY

Anti-ageing creams are expensive, so when buying keep a cool head. Beauty consultants at the counter will rationalise the cost by saying that you don't need to use very much so it only works out at 25p a day (or whatever). They will also bombard you with pseudo-scientific jargon. Here are some of the terms you will hear when you start talking about anti-ageing creams:

Liposomes Tiny spheres of fat which carry 'biologically active' ingredients, capable, so it's claimed, of passing through the dead cell barrier and merging with the outer membrane of living cells, whereupon they discharge their ingredients plus some water. They have a time release action which ensures that any moisturising effect lasts throughout the day (Estée Lauder's Future Perfect gel claims to moisturise skin for up to eighteen hours).

Retinyl Palmitate A vitamin A derivative, and a newly trumpeted addition to skin creams ever since Retin-A made its debut as a wrinkle reverser. There is, apparently, a chance that this *can* break down in the skin and as a result work in a similar though less dramatic way to Retin-A.

Collagen The molecules of collagen are too big to penetrate the skin and affect the collagen of the dermis. However, collagen *is* acknowledged as a useful ingredient in moisturising creams because it bonds very efficiently with the dead cell layer.

Free Radical Scavengers Anti-oxidants Body metabolism and ultra-violet light both trigger the release of free radicals. These are molecules of oxygen which attach themselves to the molecules of other cells and bring about disorganisation of their DNA. This leads to the gradual disintegration of body tissues which we regard as a normal part of ageing. The theory goes that if we can neutralise free radicals before they have a chance to do their dirty work, then we can stay younger, look younger, for longer. Our food provides free radical scavengers in the notable form of vitamins A, C and E (this, incidentally, is why smoking uses up so much vitamin C). However, some doctors and scientists are sceptical that vitamins can enter the skin let alone affect this process, and no scientific evidence exists in its support. Vitamin E is included in many cosmetic creams because it has anti-oxidant properties that make it a good preservative.

RETIN-A

'If I had to choose between Retin-A and my husband, Joe would have to go.' So one woman enthused to an American magazine. In America Retin-A has grabbed the headlines in a big way, and it's not hard to see why. The claims for this drug *are* exciting. Retin-A, it appears, can do marvellous things to sun-damaged skin, improving texture and tone, and noticeably softening fine lines. Many users report rosier, smoother and yes, younger looking skin.

WHAT IS RETIN-A?

Retin-A (also known as retinoic acid or tretinoin) is a derivative of vitamin A (retinol) and comes in cream, gel or liquid form. It was Dr Albert Kligman of the University of Pennsylvania who first established its usefulness as a treatment for acne back in the late sixties. Over the years some of his patients, in particular middle-aged women, noticed it had rejuvenating effects too, and remarked on their smoother, less wrinkled skin. Kligman, sceptical at first, eventually confirmed their observations with clinical trials and the legend of Retin-A, as a medical treatment for skin ageing, was born.

Retin-A is first and foremost a drug, and as such has deep and far-reaching effects on the skin. As a treatment for sun-damaged skin its action is still under close medical scrutiny, but research so far suggests that it works in the following ways:

☀ *Retin-A stimulates the cells* in the epidermis to turn over more rapidly. The epidermis actually starts to thicken, so the skin looks a little plumper.

☀ *At the same time* dead cells on the surface of the skin (stratum corneum) thin out and compact together, so skin looks finer and more translucent.

☀ *Increased shedding of dead skin cells* unblocks pores so they're less apparent; skin looks cleaner and smoother.

☀ *Retin-A stimulates the growth* of new blood vessels, increasing blood flow to the skin. Skin is better nourished and takes on a slightly pinker, healthier glow.

☀ *Age spots may fade* too, due to a more even distribution of melanin in the skin.

☀ *Collagen production* is stimulated which contributes to plumper looking skin. This is only noticeable, however, after long term treatment (more than one year).

Retin-A delivers results – but not miracles. As Dr David Fenton, dermatologist at St Thomas's Hospital, points out, so far it only appears to work on photoaged (sun-damaged) skin. It doesn't affect the sagging or the purse-like wrinkles around the mouth that are the result of intrinsic ageing. 'British women tend to be less photoaged than their American counterparts, so although there may be some improvement it's usually nowhere near as dramatic as it's possible to achieve on skin that has been grossly aged by the sun. But there is no doubt that it does have an effect.'

Retin-A is a drug and thus only legally available on prescription from a doctor, who in turn has not received clearance from the DHSS to prescribe it for anything but acne. Ortho-Cilag, who market Retin-A worldwide, are currently engaged in research into its use as a treatment for photoageing, and the outcome of long term studies is awaited.

In the meantime don't be tempted to try Retin-A unsupervised. It has irritant side-effects which make it unsuitable for some skins, and there are plenty of dos and don'ts involved in its use. Most important of all, you must avoid prolonged sun exposure, say Ortho-Cilag, and wear a sunscreen during the day if this is possible. Retin-A does make skin very vulnerable to burning and many dermatologists advise patients to wear a sunscreen with an SPF of 15 all the time. Some studies on laboratory animals have indicated that Retin-A may speed up the appearance of sunlight-induced skin cancers. However, a report in *The Lancet* points out that so far there is no evidence that it promotes cancer in man. It is much more likely, says *The Lancet*, that regular use of the drug, especially in combination with sunscreen, would reduce the risk of some skin cancers.

Regular moisturising is another must. Skin can react to Retin-A by becoming very sore, dry and flaky indeed. And there are many cosmetics and beauty treatments which react badly on tretinoin-treated skin. Retin-A *must* be obtained from a doctor or dermatologist along with a carefully supervised regime.

Research continues apace and it's likely that one day in the future new creams based on tretinoin-type chemicals will be developed that will offer all the benefits of Retin-A with fewer of the irritant side-effects. In the meantime we can only wait hopefully and see.

SMOKING AND SKIN

If you don't smoke then you can skip this section with a light heart and congratulate yourself on your fresh, healthy complexion. If you do smoke then steel yourself and read on, *please*: you know you're behaving like a kamikaze pilot with your health and yet you *still* can't summon the motivation to stop. Maybe it will be your vanity that wins the battle in the end. No one cares why you give up, as long as you do.

Smoking is second only to the sun in its ugly and ageing effects on the skin. Many beauticians claim they can tell if a woman smokes just by looking at her skin. So can one Dr Douglas Model who, a few years ago, put the theory to the test. His results confirmed that smoking causes 'readily recognisable wrinkling and other changes to the faces of many people'. He coined the term 'smoker's face' and defined the tell-tale signs thus: lines or wrinkles on the face, particularly radiating at right angles from the lips and corners of the eyes; deep or shallow lines on the cheeks and lower jaw; a subtle gauntness of facial features, with prominence of the underlying bony contours; maybe a slight sinking in of the cheeks; a grey pigmented appearance to the skin.

There are plenty of good reasons why smoking should affect skin in this unattractive way. Nicotine constricts blood vessels so less nourishment reaches the skin and waste products are less efficiently removed. Smoking also depletes the body of vitamin C, 25mg with every cigarette. Vitamin C is vital for healthy collagen and strong capillaries. Added to this the very act of smoking – pursing your lips to hold the cigarette in your mouth, sucking in the smoke and then puffing it out – is bound to cause wrinkles in the long term. Watch yourself smoking in the mirror and you'll immediately see why you've already got the wrinkles you have, and where fresh ones are likely to appear.

Don't despair. The good news is that few of Dr Model's ex-smokers had 'smoker's face'. On this point his conclusions were cautious: either they had never had smoker's face, or they'd put on some weight and puffed out their cheeks so the wrinkles were camouflaged or – and this is the theory we would like to believe – their 'smoker's face' had simply disappeared. Stop smoking now and watch your skin blossom day by day.

THE HOLISTIC APPROACH TO SKINCARE

A well-balanced diet, adequate sleep, regular exercise – these are the beauty basics that pay big dividends. Skin needs its full quota of vitamins, minerals, protein, fats and carbohydrates if it's to repair and renew itself to full potential. Exercise stimulates circulation and ensures plentiful supplies of nutrients and oxygen reach the skin. Exercise also aids sleep. When we sleep we give skin a breathing space, a chance to restore itself at maximum efficiency.

DIET

Follow all-round nutritional guidelines in Chapter Eight, but give the following vitamins and minerals celebrity billing – they're all closely related to skin health:

Vitamin C is vital for strong, healthy collagen, elastin and capillaries. It's also a powerful anti-oxidant. You will need extra supplies of vitamin C if you smoke.

Vitamin A is another important anti-oxidant. Shortage of vitamin A leads to dry, rough, scaly skin and premature ageing. Don't panic – you're unlikely to be deficient in vitamin A because the body is able to store this fat-soluble vitamin in the liver. (It's unwise to dose yourself with large amounts of vitamin A because too much can be toxic.)

Zinc. You will also need an adequate intake of zinc in order to reap the benefit of vitamin A. Zinc is necessary for collagen synthesis and wound healing. Refined food and the ageing process are just two of the factors that may conspire to lower levels of zinc in our bodies. Supplements can be useful.

Selenium is a trace element and an anti-oxidant that pops up in many anti-ageing supplements, although there is very little available evidence at the moment to suggest it does have any important function. Find it in eggs, tuna fish, brewers' yeast and kelp.

Essential Fatty Acids (EFAs) have grabbed the spotlight in recent years too. EFAs help skin to retain moisture by keeping cell membranes fluid and flexible. Although they're widely available in everyday foods there are many factors that can prevent EFAs from being properly utilised by the body, for instance, trans fatty acids found in cooking oils, margarine, sweets and bakery products all inhibit absorption, as can stress, the ageing process and virus infections. Evening Primrose Oil contains EFAs in a form that can be easily and efficiently assimilated and for this reason is taken by many people to improve skin condition, either in capsules by mouth, or applied directly to the skin in oil form. EFAs (sometimes known in cosmetic – but not medical – circles as vitamin F) are an increasingly popular ingredient in skin creams too, although evidence is conflicting about their efficacy.

Of course many other vitamins and minerals play an important part in keeping skin in optimum condition – there's simply nothing to beat a well-balanced diet if it's good skin you're after.

EXERCISE

Just as smoking impairs circulation to the skin, so exercise increases it, and research shows that the effects are nothing but beneficial. In some studies long term, regular exercisers were found to have thicker dermises, fewer wrinkles and less sagging than their more apathetic sisters. Aerobic exercise is the key because it really gets the blood pumping. Massage is a gentler but nonetheless useful way to improve circulation to the skin and you can do this every day as you apply and remove cleansers and smooth moisturiser into your skin. Don't do it vigorously though, or it may have the reverse effect and damage skin instead. Move up the face, using circular movements with the finger pads, in a slow and leisurely fashion.

SLEEP

You don't have to be particularly observant to notice the ravages exacted on the face when you're tired and short on sleep. Muscles droop, circulation slows down, skin texture suffers. Skin cell renewal and repair is at its most vigorous between the hours of 1 am and 4 am so beauty sleep is not a myth. The amount of sleep a person needs is as individual as a fingerprint. If you need eight or nine hours to look and feel at your best, then move heaven and earth to ensure that's how much you get.

DO YOU NEED A NIGHT CREAM?

Your skin is the best judge of that. Very dry skin may well need an extra moisturising boost at night, but a thick layer of cream isn't necessary. Rich, heavy creams may induce blackheads. Monitor your skin with and without – just check how it looks after two weeks' use.

A FEW WORDS ABOUT EYE CREAMS

Heavy creams can make the under-eye area puffy. Use fine, light creams only. Eye gels are very popular, but some can have a perverse drying effect if used regularly.

FACIAL EXERCISES

Should you or shouldn't you exercise the muscles of your face? Those who believe you shouldn't argue that facial muscles get enough exercise anyway and contorting the face further only hastens the onset of expression lines. They are, however, probably outweighed by those in favour, some of whom claim that facial exercises are the next best thing to a face-lift.

The trick with facial exercises is not to indulge in any that over-stretch and wrinkle the skin unnecessarily. There are those who believe the skin should barely move at all.

We would all benefit from learning how to relax the horizontal creases in our forehead and the vertical lines between brows. First massage away furrows with the palm of your hand, moving up the forehead to the hairline. Hold for a count of three and then repeat several times. Now open your eyes wide and raise your eyebrows; let your eyebrows drop but try to maintain the relaxed state of your forehead. Do these exercises looking in the mirror at first. Learn how it feels when your forehead is not creased into lines and try to recreate this sensation whenever you can throughout the day.

BLEMISH BUSTERS
MOLES
Concentrated clumps of pigment cells, varying in size and usually found all over the body. There's no cause as such: we're born with our moles and they stay with us for life. In most cases they are quite harmless. However, there is a connection between moles and some forms of skin cancer so if you notice any changes in a mole, e.g. sudden increase in size or bleeding (and it's worth taking care when you're having a bath to check them out regularly), it is important to visit your doctor immediately.

Treatment
Unsightly moles, on the face for example, can be removed by minor cosmetic surgery. The mole is removed by excision (i.e. it is literally cut out) usually under a local anaesthetic. There will be a few stitches – often just one or two, depending on the size of the mole. A dressing is worn afterwards and the stitches are removed in five to six days. The incision will heal in two to three weeks, and scars will fade over four to six weeks.

With any pigmented skin condition it is important to make your first port of call your doctor. The surgery itself must be carried out by either a plastic surgeon or a dermatologist. If the mole is in an unsightly position on your face and is causing you distress or discomfort you will be eligible to have it treated under the NHS, but waiting lists may be long. The alternative is to have private treatment with referral from your GP. At the time of writing mole removal costs in the region of £100, including consultation and tests on skin tissue.

You will be left with a tiny scar, slightly wider than the mole itself. Discuss this with your specialist.

BROKEN BLOOD VESSELS ON THE FACE AND LEGS
Blood capillaries near the surface of the skin that are permanently dilated due to weakness of the vessel wall or slackness in supportive tissue. They can be an inherited condition or the legacy of sun damage. Extremes of temperature and alcohol may aggravate the condition by increasing blood flow.

Treatment
There are two methods of treatment: one is a form of electrolysis which cauterises the blood vessels; the second, called schlerotherapy, involves injecting a chemical into the capillary to shrink and collapse it.

Electrolysis An electrolysis needle is inserted along the capillary at various points and a small electric current passes through the needle generating just enough heat to cauterise the vessel and dry up the blood. Sometimes further treatments are needed to do the job thoroughly. However, it is not unusual for the capillary eventually to refill with blood, or for new red veins to appear.

If you plan to have your broken blood vessels treated by electrolysis it's vital to find an experienced operator. Some members of the British Association of Electrolysists have earned a special diploma in red vein treatment. It may be possible to find a dermatologist who is willing to offer this on a private basis. Ask your doctor for advice and/or referral.

Schlerotherapy The capillary is injected with a chemical solution that sets up an inflammatory reaction causing the capillary walls to shrink and close up. Some capillaries may have to be re-treated, but it's suitable for both face and legs.

Schlerotherapy is a medical treatment and the solution used is available on prescription only. You'll have to shop around to find a beauty salon or cosmetic surgery clinic who can call on doctors or nurses to offer this service. Schlerotherapy was pioneered by a nurse called Katherine Corbett and many women make the pilgrimage to London to have their veins treated by her.

SKIN TAGS

Protuberances of loose fibrous tissue (like mushrooms on stalks). They may be brown, pink or flesh-coloured and are most commonly found on the neck, around the underarm area and sometimes the face. They vary in size. There's no known cause but they are associated with the ageing process.

A popular beauty salon treatment for skin tags is to cauterise or coagulate them by electroloysis, using an electric current passed through a fine needle. The needle is inserted several times all over the tag and a short burst of mild current heats it up and coagulates the skin tissue. Larger skin tags on pronounced stalks are sometimes cauterised at the base with a slightly stronger current. In one fifteen-minute session an experienced electrolysist may be able to deal with up to twenty skin tags.

Always check with your doctor before seeking beauty salon treatment for skin tags. If they're very unsightly or are constantly getting snagged and becoming infected you may be eligible for treatment under the NHS. Either way a reputable electrolysist working within a beauty salon should always ask for a GP's letter before proceeding.

FACIAL HAIR

From their twenties onwards many women notice a dark shadow of hair on their upper lip, and sometimes the hairs grow stronger and darker after the menopause when oestrogen levels drop.

Treatment Although it's perfectly normal, facial hair can be embarrassing and most women cope with it on a do-it-yourself basis. Try *bleaching* first.

There are plenty of facial bleaches on the market to choose from: follow the instructions carefully and if the end result isn't pale enough (i.e. if the hair is left an orangey or yellow shade) try another application of bleach a few hours later. Facial *depilatory creams* will remove the hair quickly and easily but there are snags. Hair is removed from just beneath the surface of the skin so regrowth comes through quickly and all at once, with the net result that the skin feels rough and stubbly, sometimes just a few days after treatment. Never be tempted to shave. This thickens up the surface of the skin and coarse stubbly regrowth is a daily problem.

Do-it-yourself removal is a constant headache. There's only one way to remove hair permanently and that's with electrolysis. This works by destroying the blood vessels at the root of the hair with heat, so they are rendered incapable of nourishing new hair growth.

An ultra-fine needle is slipped down the hair follicle until the root of the hair is reached (this shouldn't hurt). Then a minute electrical current passes down the needle and cauterises the hair root (you will feel a slight tingling or burning sensation for a few seconds). The hair is then removed with tweezers. The length of treatment time builds up slowly from five to ten or fifteen minutes as your pain tolerance levels increase (some people find it more unpleasant than others) and sessions are usually spaced at weekly or fortnightly intervals. There will be some reddening of the skin afterwards and occasionally a small scab will form (this means your skin has been burnt and it shouldn't happen often; if it does, don't go back to the salon for any more treatment). Sometimes a hair will have to be treated several times before it is killed off and there will always be some hair not visible because it is in the process of growing through. When it does eventually appear it may be mistaken for regrowth. The snag is that an area like the upper lip can take from six to eighteen months to treat completely so it takes determination to stay the course.

Again it's vital to find a skilled and experienced electrolysist.

WHITEHEADS OR MILIA
Tiny, hard, pearly lumps which often form on the cheekbones or around the eyes. They are small cysts of keratin and waste matter which build up around the mouth of a pore. Fair skins are particularly prone to whiteheads and they seem to be associated with prolonged sun exposure. Take yourself along to a good beauty salon and they will probably steam them first and then nick the top with an electrolysis needle so the contents can be eased out. Don't try this yourself. If the whiteheads keep coming back cover them with a concealer cream.

BLACKHEADS
They are often permanent fixtures around the nose where pores have become widened after years of congestion with sebum. The only thing to do is to try to keep pores clear by thorough cleansing – scrub creams will help. Beauticians are very adept at squeezing out blackheads, in fact it's an

important part of every facial. They usually do it manually, having thoroughly steamed and softened the area first. The only trouble is that the blockage nearly always forms again – you have to engage in an ongoing campaign against blackheads.

COSMETIC CAMOUFLAGE

Many skin problems including scars, birthmarks, broken veins, vitiligo (patches of white on the skin where there is no pigmentation) can be successfully covered with special camouflage make-up. With the right products and expert application, superb results can be achieved. Innoxa have a range of make-up called Keromask which is available from Innoxa consultants in some department stores and branches of Boots. Veil Cover Cream made by the Thomas Blake Co., based in Yorkshire, is also excellent. It is often necessary to blend together two or three creams in order to achieve a precise match with skin colour, and applying them correctly is important too. The Red Cross operate a camouflage advisory service in many hospitals. Contact your GP for a letter of referral or write to Rita Roberts, British Red Cross Society, 9 Grosvenor Crescent, London SW1X 7EJ (please enclose an SAE).

STRETCH MARKS

There's no easy solution to the problem of stretch marks. They are the legacy of rapid weight gain, and high levels of the hormone progesterone in the body. Some women are left with stretch marks after puberty or pregnancy. They occur when the elastin fibres deep in the dermis rupture. Once this has happened you can massage the skin with a myriad of expensive oils and potions till you're blue in the face but nothing will repair them. A 'tummy tuck' which removes excess skin on the abdomen will get rid of any stretch marks in this area too. Apart from this the only preventive measure you can employ is to avoid excessive weight gain.

DARK CIRCLES UNDER THE EYES

As we get older so the skin all over our body begins to thin, but under the eyes, where skin is very thin anyway, this sometimes reveals underlying blood vessels and gives the impression of reddish-blue circles. The skin here can become more heavily pigmented than the rest of the face and sometimes bone structure emphasises the dark, shadowy effect.

If you've never had dark circles before and suddenly develop them out of the blue it's best to see your doctor: constipation, anaemia or a nutritional deficiency are possible causes. Plenty of sleep, exercise and a high fibre diet may help; if not then you'll simply have to resort to camouflage with a concealer cream.

HANDS

Hands betray age alarmingly. Skin becomes loose and slack and sometimes peppered with freckles known as liver or age spots. You may be surprised to learn that it is possible to have excess skin on the hands excised by plastic surgery, or planed down by means of dermabrasion (another plastic surgery procedure), so it grows back firmer and fresher and tighter.

To prevent age spots always wear a high factor sunscreen on your hands when out in the sun. Protect them from rough treatment with gloves of all descriptions: gardening gloves, washing up gloves, white cotton housework gloves, warm winter gloves. Place hand cream at strategic points around the house and use it lavishly as often as you can. It's impossible to pamper hands too much.

FEET
It has become a cliché to say that painful feet cause wrinkles but as with most clichés there's more than a grain of truth behind it. Painful feet lead to a pained expression on the face and militate against a youthful spring to the step. It's also very difficult to exercise effectively if your feet hurt. Corns and bunions are the direct result of tight, ill-fitting shoes. Corns should be dealt with by experts. In fact a regular session at the chiropodist's could turn out to be one of the most rewarding beauty treatments you ever give yourself. You'll feel as though you're walking on air afterwards. Bunions can be nipped in the bud by wearing correctly fitted shoes; your chiropodist may be able to suggest helpful exercises. As a last resort surgery may be necessary.

Prevent callouses from building up by rubbing away hard skin with a pumice stone or metal file (especially designed for the job) when you're in the bath.

THE BODY BEAUTIFUL
The beauty of body skin is that it responds so quickly and gratefully to any pampering it receives. Less sensitive and temperamental than the facial kind, you can, frankly, be more brutal with body skin and thus achieve faster results.

Body skin may have been shamefully neglected over the years but it's probably in surprisingly good condition thanks to almost year round protection from ultraviolet light. However, there are certain zones that don't respond to neglect with as much good grace as the rest. Give them top priority.

✺ **Start at the top with your neck.** This should of course have a place in your daily skincare routine, but for some reason usually doesn't. The neck shows age much faster than the face – there's less fat and fewer oil glands here – and it suffers a lot more mechanical wear and tear. Just stop and think for a moment how often you move your neck around in the course of a day. Necks are also quick to reflect bad posture and fluctuations in weight. Soap and water cleansing in the bath, plus non-existent moisturising, soon result in coarse-textured grey-looking skin, reminiscent of a plucked chicken. If cleansing your neck as well as your face is certain to prove too much for you (because it's a messy business), take a different tack. Slather your neck with cream or lotion (any old cream or lotion will do) before you step into the bath. Then simply wash it off after a few minutes with soap and water. Face packs, exfoliating creams and lavish moisturising will all help enormously too. Give your neck a real treat at least once a week.

✺ *Skin on the chest* is very thin and fragile and can develop a 'cigarette paper' look, due to years and years of sun exposure. A daily, gentle application of fine oil will help here: try chamomile aromatherapy oil (diluted first) or Evening Primrose oil. A good supportive bra is a must to avoid further dragging and stretching of this delicate area, and of course a sun block must be worn from now on when you're out in the summer sun.

✺ *Backs* suffer from the opposite problem – the skin is much thicker here and there are more sebaceous glands than anywhere else on the body. Even at the advanced age of forty your back may still be greasy and prone to the odd spot. Wake up skin with a body brush made from natural fibres and use it *dry*, skimming lightly over the back to zip up circulation and remove dead skin cells. In the bath give it a jolly good scrub with a loofah or bath mitt and plenty of lather and make up a final rinse with fresh water and a tablespoon of cider vinegar.

✺ *Elbows, heels and knees* can end up as dry and leathery as old crocodile skin if you're not careful. They need a more rigorous approach. A wet pumice stone on damp skin is the time-honoured remedy, but a bit too barbaric for our taste. Try vegetable oil and granulated sugar instead. Mix one teaspoon of each in the palm of your hand and then massage vigorously into skin. Wash off with soap and water.

All over body buffing and polishing takes place in the bath. Lock the bathroom door and allow yourself at least half an hour of unadulterated privacy and bliss. There are many wonderful ways you can pamper your body and relax your mind, it's just a question of how imaginative or creative you want to be.

A major chore at bathtime will be to remove dead skin cells and sand down gooseflesh (accumulations of dead cells that have hardened around hair follicles). You must decide which method of exfoliation you want to use and then stick with it, make it a familiar bathtime friend. Choose from loofahs, body brushes with natural bristles, rough cloths or scrub creams. Then prepare for a beautifying bath.

Beautifying baths are never hot, which dries out the skin horribly and makes you weak and tired. (Remember, the cooler the bath, the more energising it will be.) And they rarely contain bath foam. Bath foams are only useful if your skin is oily, because they're very drying.

Some of the best baths contain a tablespoon or two of vegetable oil (e.g. sunflower or almond oil) or a fragrant bath oil, to lubricate the skin. But there's no need to stop here; shop around and you will find that there are many other interesting bath additives to be found – choose from seaweed baths, mud baths, milk baths, herbal baths and aromatherapy baths. Less exotically you could use Epsom salts to create an invigorating bath, or add cornstarch to soften hard water and smooth the skin.

A beautifying bath is always rounded off with a generous application of body oil or lotion. This must be massaged in all over, so that every inch of skin is covered.

SIX

Wake Up Your Make-Up

'Most women are not so young as they are painted.'
Max Beerbohm, A Defence of Cosmetics, 1922

Jenny makes up every day in ninety seconds flat using the same old stuff she's been wearing since her twenties. Jane veers wildly between no make-up at all and wearing too much. 'I just can't seem to get it right any more,' she wails. 'I look washed out when I don't wear it, and older when I do.'

Jenny's lucky because the make-up routine that she honed to perfection in her twenties was so simple that it still suits her today. But Jane – well, Jane is definitely going through a Mid-Life Make-Up Crisis.

It can happen to anyone. One minute your make-up does its usual trick of transforming you into a sultry-eyed, glossy-lipped beauty; the next minute you're Bette Davis in *Whatever Happened to Baby Jane*. And if you've ever wondered what happened to Baby Jane, the answer is – her make-up got stuck in a time warp.

Time Warp Make-Up is a well-known phenomenon that afflicts some of us more acutely than others. Of course if you don't wear make-up then it won't afflict you at all, but if you do then as a general rule – the more you wear, the more room there is for error.

Almost all the cosmetics that were very popular in the sixties and seventies can be classified as Time Warp Make-Up, now you're forty. Black eyeliner for example (although some will dispute this hotly). Lipgloss and panstick foundation also come into this category, as do ice pink or bronze blushers and bright blue, bright green or ghoulishly purple eye shadows.

But these are just the tip of the iceberg. Technique can be a minefield too. Let's get specific. From here on in you must vow never to step outside the door again wearing any of the following . . . they're

INSTANT GIVEAWAYS

✸ *Black kohl lining the inside of your lower lashes, or anywhere else come to that.* This always was a very messy technique: under-eye smudges (inevitable) will make dark circles more pronounced. Some women do get away with it by adopting a thoroughly bohemian or wildly eccentric pose (hats help here) but on the whole its's best to exercise huge restraint with black eyeliner. It can make you look hollow-eyed and haggard and doesn't disguise lack of sparkle, merely draws attention to it. Carry on lining your eyes by all means, but do it with a soft, neutral shade, underneath the lashes, not inside them.

✸ *Fiddly eye make-up that involves three or four different eye shadows and takes a diagram to explain.* You must be terribly well organised to find the time. Everyone looks at your eye make-up and marvels, but do they notice you? Eye make-up should enhance your eyes, not attract attention away from them. Calm down, you really don't *need* all that gunk on your lids. Eye make-up these days is subtle and discreet and one-colour eyes reign supreme.

✸ *White or cream frosted eye shadow highlighting the brow bone.* It's time to wake up your make-up. It's not sleeping but in a coma. This technique dates a woman more precisely than her passport. Everyone will see your brow bone coming before they see you. Frosted white is a *brilliant* highlighter (that's the trouble) but it strikes a jarring note on any face, especially a mature one. Better by far to freshen up the brow bone area with a light application of foundation and/or powder, or a very pale version of the eye shadow that you're wearing on your lids. Peach or rose-toned blusher swept lightly across the brow bone and through eyebrows too will give a warm, cheerful boost to your face.

✸ *Powder blusher applied in a perfect stripe.* You're probably still hung up on the old sixties idea of using blusher to give shape to your face. Or you're still using the rather nasty, thin, hard brush that comes in most blusher compacts and not a nice big soft one that you purchased separately and specifically for the purpose. Don't forget, blusher is supposed to make you look as though your cheeks are lightly flushed with a healthy glow. It's not a face shaper.

✸ *Outlining your mouth with brown lip liner and coating your lipstick with lipgloss.* This is straight out of the Jackie Collins school of make-up and suggests that you had your heyday in the sixties and never quite got over it. Lip pencil does a great job of defining the mouth, but it must match, or be paler than, your lipstick.

Glossy lips aren't sexy either, merely old hat. And they can get very messy and smear all over the place. If you must use gloss, restrain yourself to just a touch in the centre of your lower lip.

✸ *Pearlised or frosted anything, i.e. foundation, eye shadow, blusher, lipstick.* Pearlised or frosted products simply don't flatter older skin. They make it look worse – more crépey, more crinkled, more open pored. Stick to matt, semi-matt or creamy products instead.

✸ *Tan foundation.* This won't fool anyone you've just come back from the West Indies – they'll just think you're wearing tan foundation. Tanned foundations are a cliché; there are much cleverer ways to look summery these days. Try a fake tan product designed for the face, bronzing gel or tinted moisturiser instead.

✸ *Heavy eye make-up, strong blusher and bright lipstick all worn at the same time.* Don't do this unless you're Joan Collins, or auditioning for a part in *Knots Landing*. You can't emphasise *everything* without looking desperate or clownish or both. Stick to the rules no matter how tempted you are to break them: if you're going to wear bright lipstick go easy on the eye make-up and vice versa. Blusher should *always* be subtle.

✸ *Fake freckles, blusher swept across the bridge of the nose, shading techniques designed to slim the nose, minimise double chins or hollow out cheeks.* Most of the so-called face-shaping tips and tricks of the sixties and seventies were conceived in the photographic studio – and quite frankly that's where they should have stayed. You simply can't get away with complicated shading techniques in the harsh light of day, and this is certainly no age at which to start trying.

WHAT TO AIM FOR NOW

It's time to put the past behind you and accept that fortysomething make-up demands a fresh approach.

Certain facts must be faced. Number one is that you've changed. You don't look quite the same any more. Your face shape has fined down, your skin tone is paler, your lip line has softened and your eyes have an interesting world-weary look about them. Is this really such a bad thing? Your face has more character now – you probably look better than you did when you were a bland, plump-faced girl of twenty. You actually don't *need* heavy make-up any more. Okay, so you have a few wrinkles. So do your friends. So do film stars and great beauties. Forget about wrinkles. Foundation isn't Polyfilla, it can't fill them in. But it can – if you wear the wrong kind – accentuate them.

Make-up is a useful prop now, nothing more, nothing less. It can cheer up a tired face, and add a dash of glamour to a dressed-up look. But it's not capable of effecting heavy disguise. It never was – it's just that when we were young everyone expected us to look ridiculous from time to time so no one commented when we did.

The trick now is to wear the least make-up to the best effect. The look you need is light and polished, defined and skilful.

To get it right you will probably have to experiment a lot at home in front of the mirror. You will probably have to devise a whole new colour scheme for your face: one that works with your natural colouring, not against it. Colour Analysis may help here. The right shade of lipstick and blusher can have a magical effect, fast-forwarding the face into flattering soft focus, so it's worth persevering.

Invest in the very latest high-tech foundations for a light silky finish. Spend a fortune on eye shadows. This is worth it for the wide choice of subtle shades available in the top ranges, which retain their colour on your lids and last. You can be as mean as you like with everything else. It's really not worth bankrupting yourself just to brandish designer packaging in the ladies' loo.

Arm yourself with all the tools of the trade. You may have resisted making this kind of serious commitment to make-up till now, but think of them as time and money savers and enjoy the expertise they'll help you to acquire. You'll get the very best value from your make-up if you apply it correctly, and it *is* much easier to blend eye shadows and blushers in a subtle fashion if you do it with a top quality brush. Minimum requirements include: a thin wedge of synthetic sponge for applying foundation, a flat ¼ inch brush for eye shadow, two fine tapered eyeliner brushes (one for eyeliner, one for concealer), a large soft brush for powder blusher and an even larger one for loose powder, and an old toothbrush for brushing through brows.

LIGHT IS EVERYTHING

It's more important than ever to make up in strong true light. Light can play tricks with the forty-year-old face, flattering you hugely one minute and exposing you cruelly the next.

When making up it is sensible to err on the safe side. Harsh lighting won't do much for your morale, but at least you'll get a clear picture of what you really look like and will be able to avoid embarrassing mistakes. Don't make up under fluorescent lights ever, if you can help it, because these drain colour from the face so you're tempted to put more on. Don't make up with the light behind you either – it's far too soft and flattering. Find a place to make up where the light streams straight towards your face; electric light should hit your face from the sides, not above, which throws shadows.

Here, then is a step-by-step make-up plan. Everything you need to know, from shopping for your make-up in the first place to how to use it once you've bought it, plus every trick in the book to get maximum mileage from your new, pared-down routine.

STEP ONE: HOW TO FAKE FLAWLESS SKIN

Cheaper than a face-lift, clever camouflage can even out skin colour, cover imperfections such as broken veins, blotchiness and under-eye shadows, refine skin texture and provide a smooth base for blusher, eye shadow and lipstick.

The smart approach now is a flexible one, one that doesn't necessarily involve wearing foundation all over your face every day. The idea is to invest in three basic products – concealer cream, foundation and powder – and then juggle them cleverly to fit your mood requirements and schedule.

Forget all those out-worn ideas about turning your face into a blank canvas – make your camouflage kit work for you in a much more subtle way. Here are some options you might like to try.

❋ *Use foundation only* on the parts of your face that need some help: usually nose, under eyes and maybe across the cheeks. Blend carefully. Optional: follow with an all-over dusting of loose, translucent powder.

❋ *Apply concealer cream* to cover imperfections (e.g. blackheads around the nose, red veins, dark circles) and then powder over entire face lightly.

❋ *Settle for just powder alone.* Use pressed powder for more coverage, loose powder for less. Or invest in one of the new pressed powder-and-foundation combinations. They look like ordinary pressed cream powder but are much, much silkier. Smooth them on with a sponge and you'll enjoy the coverage of a foundation, the lightness of powder. Brilliant!

THE ART OF CONCEALMENT

Concealer creams, those faithful friends of our spotty youth, should now zoom into new importance. Take them seriously because they can do just as much as foundation to lift a tired face.

Concealer creams come in all shapes and forms these days: sticks, compacts, tubes with sponge-tipped applicators. There are even some mousse concealers around too. The first two offer more coverage but the thinner, runnier ones are popular because they don't sit so heavily on the skin. However, the stick kind needn't feel heavy if you apply them properly.

Look for a shade slightly lighter than your skin colour/foundation. 'Slightly', though, is the operative word. If it's too pale you'll be into circus territory again, and look like a clown.

How to apply

Expert application is the key, so follow closely. You can wear concealer under or on top of foundation, or on its own. We reckon the last two options are best.

First study your face in the mirror carefully and look for areas of dark shadow or red veins that need concealment. You'll find this extremely helpful and revealing.

Never put concealer cream straight on to your skin from stick or pot. *Always, always, always* put a dab on to the back of your hand first and then with a fine brush (e.g. eyeliner brush) take up a little and paint it on to the shadowy area *only*. This sounds finickity, but I promise it isn't. If you put too much concealer on (which you're bound to do if you don't follow this advice) then you'll have to smear it over a large area to get rid of it, and there you'll be with thick patches of make-up everywhere and all subtlety gone. Once you've got this minute amount of concealer on your skin, press and pat it into your skin with a light touch. Don't blend. Then add a little more concealer if you need it and so on. Finish with a light dusting of powder.

Areas most likely to benefit from artful concealment: red veins on the cheeks or around the nose, dark skin under and around the eyes, any shadowy area. Concealer creams can't camouflage lines or wrinkles, but may help to soften nose-to-mouth furrows (choose the lightest texture and use the lightest touch for this kind of job).

In the case of eye bags, don't put concealer all over the baggy area; this will simply highlight the bags and bring them forward. Instead apply concealer *underneath* the bags, in the ledges that throw shadows.

SHOPPING FOR FOUNDATION

Adopt a big spender approach. This is a major investment and the more expensive brands do seem to give a finer finish, more coverage and longest-lasting results. Start by looking at top-of-the-range stuff – brands like Clinique, Estée Lauder and Elizabeth Arden all have a flawless record in this department and are favoured by the professionals.

Your first decision will be which formulation, and this is usually keyed into skin type (i.e. are you oily, dry or a bit of both?). Over forties must avoid heavy formulations which settle into lines and wrinkles and make them look worse.

Setting out on your shopping expedition for foundation you will soon find yourself overwhelmed by the vast array on offer. This is why you must skim through our Essential Guide to Foundation first. Forewarned is forearmed.

FOUNDATION TO BE WARY OF
Think twice before buying any of these:

Panstick or pancake These come in solid form. Some are greasier than others, and they're the heaviest foundations you can buy. Suitable for theatrical types only, or anyone who needs serious coverage.

Matt foundation of the creamy liquid kind They contain a lot of powder and can give some skins a dried-up, crinkly look. They're also tricky to smooth on because they dry so quickly. Test on the back of your hand first and then compare with other formulations.

All-in-one foundations These are heavy on oils, waxes and powder, the idea being you'll get substantial coverage and won't need to powder on top. Too heavy for you.

Foundations that claim to give skin a luminous glow This may just be descriptive waffle or it may mean that the foundation is frosted, in which case avoid it like the plague. Test on the back of your hand to find out which is which: there are even some tinted moisturisers which fall into this category. Frosted foundation gives older skin a heavy-textured look and maximises every pore.

FOUNDATION TO SEEK OUT
Tinted Moisturisers These defy classification: you either love them or you don't.

Those who love them rave on endlessly about how superbly well they warm up a flagging complexion thus freeing their users from the tyranny of having to wear foundation and blusher all the time. Fans also remark on how happily tinted moisturisers sit under foundation, adding a note of cheer to the proceedings.

Those who don't love tinted moisturisers complain of too little colour or too much and bemoan the lack of serious coverage – which is silly. The whole point of tinted moisturisers is the *natural* effect they bestow. Everyone is bemused as to why some tinted moisturisers come in pale, porcelain shades (answers on a postcard please).

In other words, a tinted moisturiser may or may not be the answer to a forty-year-old's prayers and the only way to find out is to try one for yourself and see.

Oil-based liquid foundation You'll be able to spot the oil-based foundation when you drip a spot on the back of your hand. It will *feel* oily and slide over a large area of skin with no trouble at all. This is one of the problems with oil-based foundations – it's very easy to use too much. When they dry you'll notice a slight shine on the skin. This is fine if it suits you, not so fine if it means you'll have to powder heavily on top to achieve a more matt effect.

Very creamy oil-based foundations (they look like double cream in the pot) can be marvellous on very dry skins, and they're thick enough to cover most imperfections too. The only proviso is that you must apply them very thinly (a damp sponge will help).

Water-based liquid foundation These are (in our opinion) top of the pops. When you apply a water-based foundation to the back of your hand you'll notice the difference: they have a thinner consistency than the oil-based kind, don't spread quite so easily and dry to a light, semi-matt sheen. They usually contain moisturisers so your skin won't feel horribly dried out either. The texture is light and fresh and just about perfect for the older skin.

Mousse foundation These are light and airy and a dream to wear. They're dead easy to apply as so little of the product actually foams out – it just seems a lot because there's so much air in there. Some leave skin with a subtle sheen so powdering on top is optional.

Oil-free foundation For oily skins only. Some are based on a mixture of alcohol, water and powders and you must shake them to blend before using. They don't give serious coverage but will even out skin colour and offer a light, powdery finish to the face. The other kind of oil-free foundation is water-based and contains silicone oils which help fix it in place and leave a matt finish.

IN SEARCH OF THE RIGHT SHADE

Your odyssey is not over yet. Having hit on the perfect formulation you must now track down the perfect shade. This must be one that matches your neck. If it doesn't there'll be a give-away tide mark at jaw level and your credibility as a sophisticated woman will be seriously in doubt.

There is a time-honoured way to embark on this quest but it does involve leaving your dignity at the front door. First you must set out for the shops not wearing foundation. Once at the beauty counters you can quickly narrow down the field by trying likely-looking foundations on the inside of your wrist. The skin here is very pale and will quickly reveal shades that are too pink, too orange, too dark. Ivory and porcelain sound entrancing but will probably make you look as white as a ghost and no one on the planet has a pink skin (any pinkness comes from underlying blood vessels showing through, not the skin itself) so anything with the merest suggestion of this shade must be discarded pronto. The truth is that flat-toned beige shades with a yellowy tinge suit most British skins best (you can go slightly darker if your skin is very pale and blotchy and needs warming up). Once you're down to one or two possible shades you must pluck up the courage and smear a little on your cheek at jawline level. Now trot out of the shop (it's impossible to make a sensible assessment under fluorescent lights) and check (using the mirror you thoughtfully slipped into your bag before coming out) how well it matches your own skin colour. Ideally it should be quite difficult to see where the foundation begins and ends. If it's an obvious blob your guess was wrong and you must keep on looking.

PUTTING ON FOUNDATION

There is, of course, more than one way to apply foundation. One popular method is to dot it on all over your face, and then blend it in at the rate of knots – if you don't the dots on your forehead and chin dry up before you can reach them.

We think it's best to apply it bit by bit, one section at a time, using either fingertips or a dry-dampened cosmetic sponge (make sure it's a very thin one though or you'll end up with more foundation inside the sponge than on your face). If you're using a water-based foundation then fingertips are best – again the sponge may soak it all up. A dampened cosmetic sponge is useful though if the foundation is thick and creamy; it's vital if you've ignored advice and are using the panstick kind. Always wet the sponge and then wring it out *thoroughly*. If it's too wet it will water down the foundation and you'll get a streaky effect.

Here then is an eminently sensible method of applying foundation:

❀ *Moisturise skin first* and then wait up to ten minutes for it to settle on the skin. Foundation slides on easier if there's some oil on the skin surface – but not too much or too little.

❀ *Dot foundation* on areas that need it most, i.e. nose and mid-cheek area. Smooth foundation all over nose and across cheeks blending out towards ears.

❀ *Now place a small dot* of foundation on the forehead, low down around the mid-point area between your eyebrows. Blend up and across towards hairline and temples. Ideally you should run out of foundation just before you reach your hairline – foundation mixed up in your hair is an icky thought. If you want to cover brow bone and eyelids with foundation (thus providing a good base for eye make-up), then use a damp cosmetic sponge in order to achieve the lightest possible film.

❀ *Finish* with a small dot of foundation on the chin, and blend out along and just under the jawbone, but never down the neck – this is too naff for words. You may have just the tiniest smidgeon of foundation left on your fingertips or sponge which you can now use to cover the upper lip area. Just the very lightest touch here, please.

Check for smears and streaks which you can smooth out with a damp sponge or fingers.

AND POSSIBLY POWDER

Powder doesn't have to look floury or frumpy – and some of us couldn't imagine life without it. It's a neat, fast way to mop up shine and looks good on its own too, straight on top of moisturised skin.

The traditional way to set foundation is with a generous application of translucent (i.e. colourless) loose powder. Well, forget the generous bit, apply it stingily instead. Your paramount aim these days is to avoid a heavy, clogging look of any description.

Dip your powder puff into the box (or if you're really up to date shake a little from your pepper pot container on to the puff) and then slap your puff against the back of your hand several times to get rid of quite a lot of the powder. Then press firmly over the areas of your face that you want to cover – maybe the centre panel only. Brush off excess with a large, soft complexion brush in a downward direction only (thus following the direction of the downy hairs on your face – apparently it can look strange if they get mussed up!).

STEP TWO: THE EYES HAVE IT

If life's too short to stuff a mushroom, it's certainly too short for fiddly eye make-up routines. There are a hundred and one other, more important things to be doing in the morning. So the first rule is: keep it as simple as possible. Better by far to have a few, swift eye-enhancing tricks up your sleeve that can be employed at a moment's notice.

Eyes still need plenty of definition, but you'll also have to work hard at giving them a fresh, sparkly, wide-awake look too. Forget the sultry smoky eye that worked so well in your youth. Heavy eye make-up using flat dark colours will make you look tired and haggard – especially if that's how you're feeling already.

First try this experiment which doesn't involve make-up at all. All you have to do is brush your brows. An old toothbrush is perfect for this. First brush your brows in the opposite direction to their natural growth, then back in the right direction again. Brush backwards once more and finish by brushing them in the right direction but with a slight upwards, outwards lift. If this has a wonderfully refreshing effect on your whole face you might like to set them in place with a soupçon of hair gel. Brows are still supposed to look quite thick and natural (not bushy though). Thin, arched shapes *are* dated, and will probably remain so for quite some time to come. If yours have been enthusiastically over-plucked for some years you could try to grow them back in, but if this doesn't work you could have a go at thickening them up with a brow brush and shadow (in a shade slightly lighter than your brows).

Always keep the brow area tidy by plucking stray hairs every day. It's particularly important to keep the area between brows clear. The brow bone may need a little attention too, but don't get carried away – only pluck hairs that are straggling away from the natural line.

The next step is to prepare the eye area with a light dusting of translucent powder or a fine layer of foundation – or both. This does such a great job of cleaning and freshening up the whole eye area that you may be able to skip eye shadow altogether after this. Mascara and liner may be all the definition you want.

The best eye shadows to use now are the boring ones. Clever make-up artists always stick to neutral colours: variations on tan, brown, grey and beige. Occasionally they go mad and add the odd touch of pink, plum or violet. Avoid any shades that overpower your natural eye colour, such as (need we say it?) bright blue, bright green, bright peach. Even some greys or navy blue can make the older eye look tired. Take care when choosing brown shades, though: dire warnings have been issued on this subject. Some browns, notably the reddy, pinky ones, can have a draining effect on women with pale, sallow complexions or grey hair. Shop for greyish, mauveish, golden-toned browns depending on your colouring, and always test on the back of your hand first. Brown has the unnerving habit of changing colour dramatically between palette and skin, and deep rich shades often turn out to be disappointingly wishy-washy when you put them on.

Ignore all pastel shades of the blue, green or lilac variety. Not flattering, decidely passé – and lilac can make your eyes look bloodshot.

If you're stuck for ideas take a close look at your eyes themselves. Note the varying shades that make up the iris and match your eye shadow to the less dominant ones.

The One Colour Eye is the modern girl's choice these days. Use your colour full strength along the lashes and then fade it out towards the brow bone. Try highlighting the brow bone with a light sweep of powder blusher in a rose or peach shade. It will cheer up your whole face.

This is no time to give up eyeliner, but you will need to refine your use of it. Black eyeliner (along with long hair and mini skirts) could be due for the old heave-ho. You may just get away with it if the line is very fine and/or you wear glasses. But do try and be objective on this issue if you can. Black is hard and unforgiving on most forty-year-old faces – so why should yours be the exception?

Look to almost any other shade but black. Grey is a good compromise, so is brown, and even sludgy greens and blues can work.

As to the eyeliner itself, choose from finely sharpened pencils that don't smudge, automatic eyeliner (gently soften with a damp eyeliner brush after using to avoid a hard line) or powder eye shadow applied with a dampened eyeliner brush. Start the underneath line at the mid point of your lower lashes and stick very close to the lashes on the upper lid. Don't take it into the inner corner of your eye unless your eyes are set very wide apart. *Soft, fine* lines only, please.

Mascara is a must of course, but curl your eyelashes first for a wide-awake look. Simply clamp an eyelash curler to the roots of lashes, hold for a few seconds and then release. Choose fibre-free mascaras for a natural silky look. Waterproof mascara is less likely to smudge but it makes lashes look hard and spiky, and hard and spiky is out, I'm afraid. One alternative is to have your lashes dyed at a beauty salon. It's relatively cheap, only needs doing every six weeks and could be a useful time-saver.

STEP THREE: BLUSH

It's a reflex action. You look pale and tired so you reach for the blusher and end up looking pale and tired but with two spots of blusher sitting clownishly on your cheeks. There's a fine line between a healthy glow and theatrical excess. Discretion is the better part of blushing. Less is *always* better than more and if you can't get it right, don't wear it at all. Try jogging every morning instead. Our friend Jane swears it puts enough colour in your cheeks to last the whole day.

But back to the affair in hand. Using blusher is trickier than ever now because the contrast between middle-aged pallor and a youthful flush is likely to be most extreme. It's time to employ every trick in the book to make blusher a more subtle affair.

Rethink first the type of blusher that you use. Cream blusher could be your best bet now: it looks more natural than the powdered kind and it's easier to blend and control (providing you don't put too much on in the first place). Mousse blusher is fabulous too and lends a light, translucent sheen to the cheeks. And there's the added bonus that you can wear this type of blusher on top of bare skin, whereas powdered blusher demands foundation and powder as a base.

Proper placement is crucial. If you don't steer well clear of your crow's-feet it looks awful; if you take blusher too near the nose the face looks pinched and narrow. Take it too far down the cheek and you're into face-shaping territory. You'll look hollow and gaunt and strange.

To apply cream blusher place three dots along your cheekbone, beginning just beneath the iris, and then blend towards the temples and just beneath the cheekbone itself.

To apply powder blusher use a large soft brush, *never* the one that came with the compact. Don't overload your brush to begin with because powder blusher is hard to control. If you do overdo it, soften the effect with lots of loose translucent powder dusted on top.

Pick light, pretty shades like coral, peach or rosy pink. Avoid burgundy (too dark and sombre) and tawny or brown shades (they can look dark, depressing and muddy on the skin).

STEP FOUR: LIPSTICK

Have fun with lipstick and wear it with as much creative panache as you can muster.

✹ **Red lipstick** is the make-up equivalent of high heels: aggressively sexy and difficult to wear. It looks fabulous on brunettes with olive-toned skin or strong-boned blondes (bleached or otherwise) but can be overpowering on the mousy brown majority. Don't give up though if it's a look you like because there are so many different shades of red around there's bound to be one that's just right for you. If in doubt compromise with a transparent shade.

✻ *Fuchsia lipstick* can look sensational too, particularly when teamed with grey hair, a cool, clear complexion and grey, white or black outfits. Again, though, strong colouring will help you to carry it off.

✻ *Orange or tangerine lipstick* makes a statement; it's not worn to flatter but to surprise. It looks best on slim, arty, *vogueish* women, wearing simple black or hot tropical shades. Hellishly difficult to wear for most of us, though.

✻ *Apricot lipstick* is tailor-made for well-groomed, silky blondes who swan about in cream or beige. Think of Meryl Streep and you've got it in one.

✻ *Peach, coral and honeyed brown shades* give a soft, warm look to the face, go with almost anything and can be adapted to see you through almost any occasion. Tone them down for a natural, healthy, outdoor look; pep them up for smart, formal or very dressy dos.

✻ *Rosy pink lipstick* always looks pretty and suits the pale-skinned brunette a treat. Again you can vary this shade to suit the mood.

Always key lipstick shades to clothes, colouring and occasion. And when wearing strong, bright lipstick be sure to get the emphasis right. More on the lips *always* means less on the eyes. In fact one of our favourite make-up look is the simplest of all: red lipstick, mascara and the finest dark line around the eyes.

There's another good reason for going to town with lipstick now. As we get older so the mouth loses some of its fullness, and the vermilion pigment which colours lips and lipline fades too. Carefully applied lipstick can do much to restore definition and give the face a more positive youthful look. Here's how to do it.

First assemble your lip colouring kit. This includes lipstick, lip pencil and lip brush.

Opt for creamy lipsticks rather than glossy ones which don't stay put for five minutes and give a messy, jam-stained look to the mouth. Long-lasting lipsticks can work well, but all too often wear off after eating and drinking and leave a vivid red stain round the mouth. Test how much staining power the lipstick has before buying by simply applying some to the back of your hand and then wiping off with a tissue. Avoid lipsticks that are pearlised or frosted: pale shades will make you look washed out and detract from mouth definition, while stronger shades translate to traffic light bright on the lips, scream artificial, and look horribly dated.

How to apply

First smear a little foundation over your mouth to act as a base and hold lipstick in place. Then, exercising due care and attention, outline your mouth with lip pencil. Choose a shade similar to or slightly paler than your lipstick. Some make-up ranges have keyed lip pencils to lipstick shades to help us get this right. Or search for a bricky shade that matches your natural lip colour exactly. Be sure to take lip liner right out to the corners of your mouth for a generous final effect. Feel free to fiddle for ages taking the lip liner just over your natural lip to give a fuller look to the mouth or just inside for a neater one. But don't get carried away; this can look sad and desperate.

Finish off by filling in with lipstick using a lip brush for accurate application and a clean line. Blot with a tissue afterwards to remove excess gunk.

FINGERTIP CONTROL

Don't bother with nail varnish unless you're extremely well organised, a lady of leisure, or find manicuring your nails a relaxing and enjoyable hobby. Nail varnish chips all the time, even if you apply it correctly, and eats up precious woman hours in maintenance. Chipped nail varnish looks awful and is a hundred times worse than no varnish at all. One could say long nails ditto except that some people have strong, sturdy nails that grow like weeds and upkeep for them is no trouble at all.

Ragged nails and overgrown cuticles look awful too, of course, and as a result are frowned upon in some circles. People *do* notice hands and judge you accordingly, although it has to be said that some are just as suspicious of perfectly painted talons as others are of unkempt ones.

Squeeze some time for nail care into your schedule if you can. Even quite short nails can be filed into a pleasing oval shape if you put your mind to it, and cuticle care is easy. Water softens up cuticles and makes them malleable so after bathing simply push them back with a towel or orange stick covered with cotton wool. (Cuticle removers tend to dry and toughen skin and should be avoided if possible.)

Buff your nails with a chamois buffer every now and again. This stimulates circulation and smooths and shines them up. Don't overdo it though or you'll end up sanding your nail away. Always keep nails clean and moisturise them frequently with cream or oil.

To make unpolished nails look special give them a French manicure. This is simplicity itself. Follow the above cuticle and buffing advice and then whiten underneath the nail tips with a white nail pencil. That's all there is to it, honestly.

If you have short, bitten nails but secretly yearn for long, painted ones, you may have toyed with the idea of sculptured nails. Think twice. Sculptured nails are very expensive and upkeep can be frighteningly so. They usually need salon attention every two weeks. Some methods involve heavily sanding your natural nails with mechanical gadgets, which for obvious reasons does nothing to improve or strengthen their condition.

However, some women find sculptured nails strong, durable, glamorous and well worth the expense and hassle. On the other hand false nails are cheaper, you can put them on and take them off yourself for nothing, and they usually come pre-painted.

Do paint your toenails. Painted toenails rarely chip, require minimum maintenance – and whenever you glimpse them they cheer you up. For this reason wear them in summer and *winter too*. Choose colours that you know you'd never have the nerve to wear anywhere else on your body: wild, exotic, shocking, fluorescent shades – whatever takes your fancy at the time.

BARE-FACED EFFRONTERY

There is, of course, another more radical alternative to all this carry-on with make-up, and that's simply not to wear it at all. Lots of women don't, including serious film actresses, right-on media folk and an encouraging number of our best friends.

There's no doubt that if you get it right the bare-faced look can work well, suggesting either a stylish *much*-less-is-more philosophy, glowing good health that it would be a crime to cover up, enviable confidence in your looks or feminist ideals.

Sometimes, however, you can't help but suspect that it suggests just the opposite; that is, you're not wearing make-up because you're so disorganised you didn't have time to put any on this morning, you're unwell, or you're very depressed about the way you look and have decided to let yourself go.

If you're keen to dispense with make-up and not have any of these rather depressing charges levelled against you it will help if you attend to a few small details first.

Number One: Maintain clean, glossy, cleverly-styled hair at all times. (Make-up can save the day when your hair looks a mess and vice versa, but to ignore both face *and* hair is risky.)

Number Two: Keep skin scrupulously fresh and clean. Dead cell debris which makes skin look lifeless and grey must be swept away daily. Wholesome food and regular exercise will help to put a healthy glow in your cheeks.

Number Three: Never neglect details. Well groomed brows are a must. Always keep stray hairs plucked or opt for the bushy-browed look – but don't straggle between the two. Keep lips well moisturised. Dried up, flaking lips (a hazard in winter) have a shrivelled look that is most unattractive.

Number Four: Cultivate a serene, relaxed or cheerful expression whenever possible. A creased, furrowed brow or anxious pursed look around the mouth gives the impression that you are uncertain or unhappy about your appearance. Natural beauties hold their heads high and look the world straight in the eye, confident in the knowledge that they look just fine.

Number Five: Never neglect general good grooming ... which has nothing to do with make-up of course. Everyone should wash her face, comb her hair and clean her teeth every day. Anything less shows lack of respect for your body and the rest of the world that has to look at you. But then you know that already.

Despite all the fighting talk make-up remains a thorny issue for some of us. Hardly surprising when you think about it – we must have been the most heavily made up teenagers in history. Brought up to believe that our eyes were 'piggy' unless heavily ringed with black, it sometimes seems that, even now, there are forty-year-old women out there who would rather die of hunger or thirst than be stranded on a desert island without their mascara. It really is time to forget all that twaddle about using make-up to minimise your bad points. You don't have any bad points. Or at least none worth mentioning. And certainly none that would be improved under a mask-like make-up. In fact it's impossible to have a healthy relationship with make-up unless you are completely comfortable about the way you look without any at all. Only then are you free to regard it with the objectivity it deserves. Enjoy wearing make-up, have fun wearing make-up, but now you're forty use less rather than more at all times. And never believe that you don't look perfectly fine without it.

SEVEN

How to Spend a Windfall:
Is Cosmetic Surgery the Answer?

'Having my breasts enlarged was the best thing I've ever done in my
life. I will have more plastic surgery . . . I'm certainly not going to
grow old gracefully – I'm going with a struggle!'
Nancy, 45

Every woman tackles the challenge of her forties in a different way. Helen celebrated her forty-seventh year with a face-lift that cost £4,000. She says it's been worth every penny.

'The money was sitting there in the bank, saved for a rainy day, and I decided this was it. I had an early menopause which left me looking much older than my years. My face just didn't match the way I felt inside. I'm a youth worker and when you deal with young people all the time you need to feel confident about yourself. I spent my mid-forties unhappy and depressed. Since the face-lift I'm a different woman. The boost to my morale has been tremendous. My teenage sons rave about it, my husband says I'm more beautiful than ever before. My self-confidence has increased by leaps and bounds.'

Helen isn't unusual. She set out for the clinics expecting to rub shoulders with the rich and famous and found instead that it's ordinary women, just like her, who fill the waiting rooms these days. Plastic surgery is still very expensive, but more women every year decide it's a price they're prepared to pay. By the end of the century the number of operations performed each week looks set to double. 'Not only will we see more women having plastic surgery,' predicts John Terry, managing director of the privately run National Hospital for Aesthetic Plastic Surgery in Bromsgrove, 'but more women will have more cosmetic surgery too. It won't be unusual for a woman to have her face-lift repeated every five to seven years.'

Cosmetic surgeon Dev Basra estimates that around 80 per cent of his patients are women in their forties. 'They begin with collagen injections, then maybe have an eye-lift, and graduate to a face-lift in their mid to late forties. Some of my patients are married to younger men, some have husbands who entertain a lot. They want to stay young and fresh looking to keep up appearances.'

'Forty is a vulnerable age,' agreed a consultant plastic surgeon at the National Hospital for Aesthetic Plastic Surgery. 'There's no doubt that there is such a thing as the mid-life crisis. The ageing process is getting established. All those years on the beach are showing their mark and gravity is beginning to exert its downward pull. Many women start to feel insecure. Their husbands may not be as interested as they used to be and although this is perfectly normal many women can't accept it. They want to feel better about themselves, they want to look better.

'Many of my patients are women who find that their breasts have become soft and shapeless after childbirth. Now their children have grown up their priorities have changed. Their social life is opening up. They've got some money and they want to spend it on clothes. So they want some padding put back in.

'And of course some families simply age faster than others. A woman may have inherited a tendency to droopy, baggy eyelids which make her look ten years older than she really is.'

Every woman has her own special reasons for submitting to the surgeon's knife. Some hit forty and find that they suddenly have both the money and the courage to deal with a problem that's been dogging them for years. And quite a few turn to plastic surgery in the hope that it will help them to retain their sharp edge in a cut-throat career. 'I didn't want to be thought of as a kindly old soul by the young women who work for me,' said Charlotte, who went on to scotch that possibility with an eye-lift, nose job and collagen injections.

Some simply want to have it all. 'I love sunbathing, smoking and drinking,' declared a glamorous, blonde businesswoman of forty-five with more than a hint of defiance in her voice, 'and I'm not prepared to give it all up in order to preserve my skin. I have collagen injections so I can carry on behaving badly without looking like an old bag at the end of it all. And yes, I probably will have a face-lift when the time comes.'

A boost to femininity often figures high on the shopping list too. Nancy swopped a flat chest for a bosomy one when she was forty-two and found it changed her entire self-image. 'I always felt very masculine before,' she says. 'Not only was I flat-chested, but my voice seemed deep, my shoulders broad, my hands big. Now I feel more feminine all over. It seems to have made my voice higher, my hands smaller, my waist tinier. Even my eyebrows don't seem so bushy!'

Few women admit to having cosmetic surgery solely to please a man and if they do, they soon discover that a good plastic surgeon will do everything he can to dissuade them. Plastic surgery doesn't save marriages or send errant husbands rushing back (and if it did, who'd want a man with such a shallow set of values anyway?). Ditch them pronto is one clinic's advice to women with husbands or boyfriends who suggest a nip or a tuck: 'We try to show them – in a gentle, sympathetic way – that these men are picking on a real or imaginary flaw in order to undermine them; and there's usually an ulterior motive behind it.'

In fact most men take the opposite tack. Helen's husband was too busy making sure she found a bona fida surgeon and avoided cowboy clinics to give much thought to the new, improved face she might achieve. Some men are so squeamish about operations they can't bear to think about the surgery involved at all. Sue's boyfriend went berserk when she told him she was having liposuction on her tummy. 'He told me he loved me the way I was,' says Sue, 'which is great but I wasn't doing it for him, I was doing it for me. He was worried and he made a big fuss, but I went ahead anyway.'

When Tina interviewed a top British soap star five years ago she was adamant that she wanted to know what she was going to look like when she grew older. 'I'd feel really cheated if a surgeon mucked it all about,' she said in feisty fashion. 'I think people worry far too much about ageing. I'm all in favour of wrinkles, they're something to look forward to!' One can't help noticing that few are rash enough to make such statements now. When the *Sunday Times* interviewed a bevy of beautiful women in their forties a few years later not one spoke out against plastic surgery. 'I'm a reasonable person,' said Jane Asher, summing up the prevailing mood in a sentence, 'so I'd have plastic surgery if I felt it was necessary.'

Our mothers never considered a face-lift because they knew their place in the world and accepted the face that went with it. Cosmetic surgery was an exotic concept in those days – and they couldn't afford it anyway. But our generation is a different kettle of fish. Middle age isn't cosy any more and we are beset by pressures at every turn. Society is still obsessed with youth and beauty and women's appearance and usually chooses to ignore those who fail to match up. And who knows where our forties will find us? Facing divorce maybe, fighting off youthful competition at work, or setting out in the world to build a new career from scratch. Some of us will be playing the dating game again, or trying to keep up with a younger man. No one can predict quite how they're going to age and if you do end up with three chins instead of two, or jowls that droop down to your shoulders – is it comforting to know that cosmetic surgery is now a socially acceptable alternative? More driving than vanity, it seems, is the need to conform. Ageism may be on the decline in our society but it still runs deep. Until we can accept and admire the older woman as she really is, lines, sagging skin and all, there will be a market for the surgical remedy.

Is cosmetic surgery a feisty approach to ageing – or a fearful one? Probably a bit of both. 'It isn't for everyone,' summed up one counsellor at a busy clinic, 'but at least women now have the choice.'

STEP BY STEP TO SUCCESSFUL SURGERY

'There's nothing safer,' says John Terry, 'than not presenting yourself for surgery and steering clear of hospitals. Women like Elizabeth Taylor talk lightly of having had "nips and tucks" when what they're really describing is major surgery. Anyone who's ever watched a breast reduction operation will know that what we're talking about here is very major surgery indeed. The breast looks as though it's been detonated by a bomb – and putting it back together again requires more skill than doing the Rubik cube three times in five minutes.'

Plastic surgery is never a step to take lightly. Even if you find a top-notch surgeon complications can – and do – occur. There is always the risk that you will react badly to the anaesthetic, pick up an infection or suffer post-operative bleeding beneath the skin if blood vessels are not properly sealed off during the operation. Your skin may not heal in a neat and tidy manner; some people develop keloid scars (Africans and Asians are most at risk); others suffer from hypertrophic scarring whereby the skin remains red and raised for a very long time (treatment with steroid creams can help). As one surgeon pointed out, 'An operating theatre is not an extension of the beauty parlour, the patient is cut and she bleeds.' Scars are the inevitable result of any operation.

Approach surgery in a sensible, level-headed way and you will help yourself to minimise some of the risks:

1. Be clear about why you want cosmetic surgery in the first place. Is it *really* necessary? If you're expecting too much or are doing it to please someone else the chances are you will be disappointed.

2. Do your homework thoroughly. Begin by reading up on the subject as much as you can.

3. Talk to as many people as you can find who have had the same surgery that you are seeking. Cross-question them closely. This is the best possible way to find out about unexpected side-effects and snags.

4. Go and see your GP once you are genned up on the subject and have, perhaps, the name of a recommended plastic surgeon up your sleeve. Talk it over and tell him the name or names you've come up with. He will be able to double-check their qualifications and may have some suggestions of his own to offer too. Your GP is a vital link in the chain because he knows your past medical history and this could be crucial to a safe conclusion.

5. Finding an experienced, skilled plastic surgeon is vital. The *Independent* newspaper now publishes a *Guide to Cosmetic Surgery*, previously only available to GPs, which lists members of the British Association of Aesthetic Plastic Surgeons. All are fully qualified in the practice of cosmetic surgery and many work as consultant plastic and reconstructive surgeons for the NHS. Make sure your surgeon is experienced in the kind of plastic surgery you are seeking. Some surgeons, for instance, do more nose jobs than face-lifts and vice versa. Just because he's good at one thing doesn't guarantee he'll be great at another.

6. You don't have to commit yourself at the first appointment. Go home and think about what's been said first.

7. Check with your surgeon what will happen if something goes wrong. If he has to re-operate find out if the cost will be passed on to you.

8. When you discuss the cost make sure that the price quoted includes surgery, anaesthetist's fee and your stay in hospital.

FACT FILE

COLLAGEN INJECTIONS

This is an effective way to soften fine lines and crow's-feet without resorting to full blown surgery. The big snags, though, are that it's temporary *and* relatively expensive.

The collagen most commonly used at the moment is an American product called Zyderm, made from cow's skin. This sounds ghastly but actually it's very similar to human collagen and is routinely used to make heart valves for surgery. When injected just beneath the skin, into the lower levels of the epidermis, it combines with the natural collagen already there and noticeably plumps up fine lines. It works beautifully on lines around the mouth, crow's-feet (but only on skin that's supported by bone, not the very fine crépey skin just beneath the eyes), forehead creases and the furrows that run between nose and mouth.

What Happens The first step is an allergy test which involves injecting some collagen into the forearm. It's been estimated in the US that three in every hundred people are allergic to bovine collagen and the reaction can be highly unpleasant, ranging from prolonged redness and swelling to shallow scarring or even, rarely, difficulty in breathing.

One month later, if all is well, the collagen is injected via a very fine needle along the lines at intervals of about one-eighth of an inch. Sometimes an anaesthetic cream is applied to the skin first to minimise discomfort and the injections themselves contain a small amount of local anaesthetic. What does it feel like? 'Little bee stings,' say most of the women we've spoken to. There will be some redness and swelling after treatment but this shouldn't last more than a day or two and then make-up can be worn.

Initially two to four sessions may be required to reach the desired effect, and then expensive top-ups are needed every six months to a year – occasionally sooner. Younger skin, or skin in good condition, will hold on to the collagen for longer. On deeper lines and wrinkles a thicker (and more expensive) form of collagen is used called Zyplast.

Some plastic surgeons or clinics will offer you Atelo collagen from Japan, which hasn't been officially licensed in Britain yet. The advantage here is that it's of a finer, more liquid consistency than Zyderm and disperses very evenly in a thin-skinned area, such as around the eyes.

Also on trial in Britain at the moment is a method of fat transferral pioneered in the States. Fat is drawn from an area such as the buttocks or thighs using a technique rather like liposuction, and then reinjected in the site that needs correction. Most surgeons agree that it's best to wait and see on this one.

What Can Go Wrong Apart from an allergic reaction to the collagen itself, in inexperienced hands the injections themselves can be wrongly placed. Costly collagen may simply be wasted if this happens, or accidentally injected into a blood vessel (you must expect some spotting of blood at injection sites in any case). Sometimes small white lumps of collagen are seen under the skin after treatment – but the great thing about collagen is that, given time, even obvious mistakes break down and disperse. Nevertheless it makes sense to choose either a plastic surgeon or a dermatologist or experienced GP for collagen treatment.

Cost This varies depending on where you go and how many tubes of Zyderm or Zyplast are used. A commercial clinic may well offer a free consultation and estimate, but charge highly for the collagen itself. If you visit a plastic surgeon you'll have to pay a consultation fee, but possibly less for the collagen. One forty-year-old woman I know has just forked out nearly

£1,000 for her initial treatment (which involved four fortnightly sessions) but is expecting to pay £250 for yearly top-ups in the future.

FACE-LIFT (RHYTIDECTOMY)

It can be hard to spot a face-lift these days because good ones look so natural. Forget the slant-eyed, scared-to-smile look of the past, the aim now is to freshen the face and firm up the jawline without over-the-top stretching of the skin and distortion of features. When friends say how well you look, assume you've been on holiday or start asking which moisturiser you're using you can be sure it's been a great success. Don't expect to look younger – hope to look 'better'.

A face-lift can't work miracles. It won't iron out every wrinkle (it would look pretty odd if it did) but it may soften some of them. It won't eradicate crow's-feet or lines around the lips. If you have a deep groove between nose and mouth (the naso-labial fold) this will be softened but not magicked away. What a face-lift does brilliantly, however, is to fight the effects of gravity, lifting sagging skin on the cheeks and neck and tidying up a jowly look at the jawline. It is often combined with an eye-lift, which corrects drooping upper lids and any bagginess underneath.

The forehead is left untouched. Many surgeons suggest treating any creases and furrows here with a follow-up course of collagen injections. A 'brow-lift' is the surgical alternative to collagen, but not always a popular option over here. Because the hairline is stretched back it increases the size of the forehead so it's not suitable for anyone with a large forehead already, and there's always the risk that you'll end up looking like Elizabeth I. 'It's an operation to be avoided,' said one plastic surgeon. 'It can leave patients with a permanently startled appearance. The scar left is just inside the hairline from ear to ear, or on the forehead itself – at its worst it can look as though you're wearing a wig or have had major brain surgery.'

How It's Done A face-lift, being a major op, is performed under general anaesthetic. An incision is made just above the temples in the hairline and travels down the front of the ear, looping upwards behind the ear (in the groove between ear and skull) and then angling backwards for two or three inches or more into the hairline of the lower scalp. Skin is separated from underlying muscle and bone, lifted upwards and backwards towards the incision line and redraped in its new position. Excess skin is trimmed away and careful stitching finishes the job. Some surgeons will tighten underlying muscles if they're very saggy – others prefer not to, claiming that a 'muscle lift' is risky (there's a slightly increased chance of permanent nerve damage), painful, and can result in an immobile, unnatural look. This is a controversial issue in plastic surgery circles at the moment – do your homework thoroughly before committing yourself to either option.

At the end of the operation drainage tubes are inserted under the skin and patients are expected to spend at least one night in hospital. If all goes well you could be home the next day, but allow yourself two weeks to rest and recuperate. Expect a swollen face and bruising at first, but this will subside faster if you apply cold compresses on a daily basis. Ears can be numb for the first three months.

What Can Go Wrong? As with any operation there's always the risk that you will react badly to the general anaesthetic, or that your skin may not heal in a neat and tidy manner. The surgeon will endeavour to make the scars in front of the ear very fine as these will be the only ones on show. In fact they usually fade to become almost imperceptible so even unswept, pulled back hairstyles can be worn.

Blood clots (i.e. haematomas) beneath the skin may form but time and/or minor corrective surgery will usually sort this out. Nerve damage is another possibility. Time is the great healer here, although some loss of sensation around the ear may be a permanent feature. Permanent damage to the motor nerves which drive the muscles of the face is rare, but has been recorded.

Cost: £2,600

More Info: Doctors don't like to predict how long a face-lift will last, but a repeat in seven to ten years is average.

EYELID CORRECTION (BLEPHAROPLASTY)
Everyone over the age of thirty develops some degree of stretched skin on her upper eyelids. If this is excessive it can result in a droopy, tired look that adds years to your age. Some people inherit a tendency to under-eye bags, which get worse as they get older. A total or partial eye-lift can work wonders, giving a brighter, younger, more wide-awake look to the whole face. It won't banish lines and crow's-feet but it will smooth them out slightly.

Correcting upper eyelid droopiness and lower eyelid bagginess are two separate procedures, although they may be carried out at the same time, often as part of a face-lift.

How It's Done Upper eyelid correction is the simpler and more trouble-free of the two operations. It can be carried out under general anaesthetic or local (with intravenous sedation to knock you out). An incision is made in the crease (i.e. socket line) of the eye and excess skin and underlying fat are trimmed away. Healing is remarkably fast if this op is done well, and stitches are removed in four to five days. Bloodshot eyes, bruising and swelling will probably see you reaching for the dark glasses for the first week. Scarring is usually very fine and fades away fast to become virtually imperceptible, particularly as it is sited in the natural crease line of the eye.

Lower eyelid correction is trickier but can be done under local anaesthetic too. An incision is made underneath the lower eyelashes and extends out into the crow's-feet area by about one centimetre. Skin is hinged upwards and forwards and underlying fat pads and excess skin are removed. It is usually only necessary to have a few stitches placed in the crow's feet area.

What Can Go Wrong One of the worst things that can happen is that the surgeon removes too much skin from the lower eyelid, so that the white of the eye beneath the iris is permanently on show. This kind of mistake can usually be resolved with a skin graft.

A more common mishap is asymmetry. Few people have perfectly symmetrical eyes to begin with and a surgeon will point this out before surgery. However, if too much skin is removed from one eye (and as one surgeon summed up, 'Every millimetre counts,') there may be an obvious difference between the two. Rough estimates have it that about one in fifteen eye-lifts have to be re-corrected.

Cost: Upper eyelids, £1,550; lower eyelids, £1,750

NOSE RESHAPING (RHINOPLASTY)

We don't usually think of a nose job as a rejuvenating technique, but according to cosmetic surgeon Dev Basra it can be just that. This is because as we get older our noses actually change. The top of the nose becomes more bulbous and the tip of the nose droops, which can make the humpy bit more prominent. Thus many people who co-existed happily with a biggish nose throughout their youth find their thoughts turning to a nose job when the mid-life crisis strikes.

As with the face-lift, fashions have changed. Forget the pert little-girl nose so favoured in the sixties (it looks silly on a middle-aged face anyway). Surgeons these days prefer to reshape a nose in a much more subtle way. It must harmonise with the lines and proportions of the face, not stick out like a sore thumb. Skin thickness determines the kind of nose you end up with too. As one clinic bluntly put it: 'A very small delicate nose cannot be made from a large thickened one.'

How It's Done Rhinoplasty is carried out under general anaesthetic. Incisions are made inside the nose so there are no external scars, although if the nostrils are narrowed too, cuts are made in the creases at the side of the nose. Bone and cartilage are delicately chiselled, underlying tissue thinned and excess skin trimmed. Usually the nasal bones themselves are fractured and reset and a plaster cast is worn for a week after the operation. Be prepared for extensive bruising and swelling around the eyes. You may have to breathe through your mouth for the first few days if your nostrils have been packed with gauze.

For the first three weeks you must restrain yourself from bending over too much, or picking your nose. Cut out sporting activities for a couple of months.

The swelling will subside eventually and you should be ready to face the world in a couple of weeks. However, it could take as long as one year (especially if you're in the older age bracket) for the nose to settle down completely to its new shape.

What Can Go Wrong Complications are thankfully rare in this most popular of all plastic surgery. Nose bleeds and infections seldom occur and can be treated simply with either extra dressings or antibiotics. Occasionally both surgeon and patient agree that the new nose shape still isn't quite right and minor adjustments are made. Few people end up with the nose of their dreams, but most are happy with the compromise.

Cost: £1,945

More Info: A nose uplift, or nose 'bob' as it's sometimes called, is another popular option and much less drastic than a full-scale nose job. In this case only cartilage inside the tip of the nose is trimmed. It works best if the tip of the nose is quite high, otherwise the natural hump of the nose becomes more pronounced. A plaster cast isn't necessary and sometimes there's no bruising at all. Patients can be in and out of hospital in half a day and back in the social swim the next morning.

BREAST AUGMENTATION
Now that couture garments demand jaunty, grapefruit-sized boobs to pad them out, breast augmentation is all the rage. By the end of the eighties over 50,000 British women were sporting silicone implants and the numbers, say the clinics, are rising fast. But not all women who have their breasts enlarged are victims of fashion. It's an operation also sought by those who've lost their shapely bust after babies; some have spent years embarrassed by a flat chest.

Breast augmentation, however, is one of the most risky of all plastic surgery procedures because it involves implanting foreign material in the body.

How It's Done This op will be carried out under general anaesthetic. The implant is usually inserted via a two-inch incision underneath the breast in the breast crease. The implants themselves are jelly-like bags – soft liquid silicone encased in a silicone envelope. More favoured by some plastic surgeons these days are polyurethane implants. They're filled with silicone but encased in a foam-like plastic material. Sometimes the implant is placed in front of the breast muscle (but behind the breast tissue), sometimes behind – opinions vary as to which is best.

After the op adhesive tapes are placed over the incision with a bra on top. Stretching and lifting is forbidden for the first few days, and even after this it's wise to go easy. Scars will take months, perhaps even a year to fade.

What Can Go Wrong Quite a lot, actually. The major problem is likely to be fibrous encapsulation – medicalspeak for the build-up of scar tissue around the implant. Breasts often go hard as a cricket ball as a result. This happens to up to 40 per cent of patients and it can strike at any time – weeks, months or even many years after the operation. The surgeon may be able to deal with this by tightly squeezing the hardened tissue with his hand until it pops apart of its own accord. Not a very decorous approach but when it works it obviates the need for further surgery.

With a polyurethane implant the risk of encapsulation is much less: some estimates have it down to 1 per cent. Although scar tissue is still laid down it embeds itself around the implant and remains soft and spongy. However, these implants are much more expensive and can be tricky to remove. They can't be resterilised either, so if one does have to be taken out, it has to be replaced with a new one. Discuss the pros and cons with your surgeon fully and get a second or third opinion if you're still not sure.

Two further risks with breast augmentation are infection and bleeding from blood vessels beneath the skin. There's always the chance that these may require further surgery.

Cost: £2,600

BREAST REDUCTION

Women who want to have their breasts made smaller, rather than larger, are a more serious breed altogether. Very large breasts can attract lots of embarrassing and unwelcome attention, and they're very heavy to carry around. Many women report back strain, rounded shoulders, collar bone deformities – and the problems don't improve with age. Katie Boyle, who had breast reduction surgery at sixty-two, and then went on TV to tell the world, admitted that when she was young she enjoyed being voluptuous, 'but they weren't so pretty when I got over the hill. They looked like pumped-up pumpkins and I ended up with a real complex about them.'

Opting for breast reduction surgery must be a carefully considered decision; the scars left behind are thicker than the hairline kind and they'll be on show when you get undressed. They do become softer, flatter and fade to a more natural skin colour in time – but this can take years rather than months. Most candidates, like Katie Boyle, are highly motivated and they're usually thrilled with the results, scars and all.

How It's Done This is major surgery and is always carried out under a general anaesthetic. The incision line, which has been likened to an anchor in shape, travels around the nipple, vertically down the centre of the breast beneath the nipple, and then curves along the breast crease towards the armpit. Skin and breast tissue are removed and the nipple has to be repositioned. You'll come round from the operation with drainage tubes inserted inside the breast and an intravenous drip to replace lost fluids. You'll probably need to spend three or four days in hospital and then go home wearing a dressing and supportive bra. There will be swelling, bruising, soreness and discomfort. Stitches are removed after two weeks.

Be prepared to lose nipple sensation completely, although you may be lucky, many are, and find that some feeling does come back. You probably won't be able to breastfeed now, either.

What Can Go Wrong Because breast reduction involves such complicated surgery there are several risks involved. One is bleeding, whereby such large clots of blood form under the skin that surgical intervention is required. Sometimes, due to inadequate blood supply during surgery, the nipple is lost completely and simply sloughs away after the operation. Reconstructive surgery is then needed to replace the lost nipple some months later, when the area has healed.

Because the scars will be on view when you're undressed any problems with healing – such as hypertrophic scarring – will add to your difficulties. Time and treatment with steroid creams will help, but it can be a lengthy business.

Cost: £2,700

More Info: Because large breasts present a physical handicap to some women you stand a better than average chance of getting this operation done on the NHS. However, waiting lists may be long, and you'll have to push very hard to get prompt attention.

BREAST UPLIFT (MASTOPLEXY)

Childbirth and the ageing process can exact a terrible toll on breasts, leaving them stretched and shapeless with all the stuffing gone. A breast uplift sounds like the magical solution – but is it? One plastic surgeon told me that a woman would have to *beg* him for an uplift before he'd go ahead. 'The scarring is considerable. I'd rather do an augmentation first and then if she's not happy with that, discuss the possibility of an uplift. But it is a more complicated operation and a woman must be fully prepared for the scarring involved.'

In fact a breast uplift leaves you with much the same scarring as a breast reduction does, but it's less radical surgery because no breast tissue is removed, just excess skin. There is less likelihood that nipple sensitivity will be affected too, and you'll probably be able to breastfeed afterwards – although it makes sense to wait till your childbearing days are over before spending money on an uplift.

Cost: £2,600 upwards

TUMMY TUCK (ABDOMINOPLASTY)

Don't be fooled by the tummy tuck tag – this definitely comes into the 'major operation' category. The aim is to remove loose flabby skin and tighten slack muscles; it's not a cure for obesity because excess fat is not removed. In fact the surgeon will insist that you're as near as possible to your ideal weight to start with, and advise you not to put on weight afterwards. One welcome side-effect of a tummy tuck is that in the process of exercising excess skin some stretch marks may be snipped off too.

How It's Done This operation is always performed under general anaesthetic. The incision line is positioned low, just above the pubic hair, and runs from hip to hip. The aim is to leave you with a scar that can be hidden by knickers or a bikini bottom.

A triangular area of skin and underlying fat is removed and skin from the upper abdomen is drawn downwards to meet up with the point of incision. In the process muscles are tightened and the navel repositioned too.

Budget for a slow recovery: three days in hospital, three weeks resting at home, six weeks before it's safe to do anything strenuous. This is not a painless operation: 'agony' is how one woman described the post-op sensation. Nevertheless you'll be expected to get up and walk on the very first day, even though you'll only be able to manage it in a 'bent double' position because your stomach will feel so tight. Daily exercise of the gentle kind is vital, though, to keep the circulation going and prevent deep vein thrombosis in the legs. Expect swelling and numbness in the lower abdomen for a few months, maybe even a year.

What Can Go Wrong Scars will remain red and raised for quite some time; allow eighteen months to two years for them to settle down completely. Repositioning the navel is tricky and sometimes during the operation blood supply is cut off and it's lost completely. Fashioning a new one is usually no problem.

Cost: £2,700

LIPOSUCTION

Liposuction vacuums out fat from beneath the skin, so it sounds like a short cut to weight loss. Not so. You must be at your ideal weight beforehand – in fact your plastic surgeon will insist on it. Liposuction removes stubborn, localised areas of fat left behind after dieting. Jodphur thighs, thick ankles, a bulging tummy or a double chin (liposuction is often used to remove a double chin as part of the face-lift procedure) – these are all prime candidates for treatment. The younger you are, the better the outcome is likely to be because skin must be elastic enough to spring back into shape once the fat has been removed. In fact once the fat cells are removed they can't regenerate so the results are deemed permanent – unless you gain a lot of weight.

How It's Done Liposuction is performed under a general or local anaesthetic. A small (less than one centimetre) incision is made in the skin (in a natural crease line if possible) into which a long metal tube is inserted. This is then moved around under the skin, hoovering out the fat which in turn is sucked through a tube and into a cylinder. The treated area is firmly bandaged for at least one week. Expect to look badly bruised afterwards and prepare for some pain and discomfort – although this varies in intensity from person to person.

What Can Go Wrong If liposuction is badly done then the skin can be left with a lumpy, corrugated look which may be worse than the fatty area it was meant to improve. It's vital to choose a surgeon skilled in this procedure.

Cost: £1,875

CASE HISTORY

Nancy, forty-five, had a breast augmentation done when she was forty-two. She is divorced, runs her own successful hairdressing business and lives alone in London.

'Before the operation I don't think a day went by when I wasn't unhappy with myself. I was completely flat-chested, I had no breasts at all, just nipples. I'd try on clothes and think, God, I look terrible. I was always buying expensive tops to hide the fact that I didn't have a bust, and the beach was a nightmare. There I'd be all rigid and hunched up in a bathing suit, never a bikini, hardly daring to walk across the beach and down to the sea.

'I never thought of plastic surgery. It never crossed my mind until I was in my early forties, and one of my clients came into the salon and said, 'Nancy, I've had my boobs done, I've had them made bigger!' And there she was in a low-cut summer dress with a cleavage for the first time! She was so proud of them that she stripped off so I could have a proper look. Well, they looked great, and I couldn't see any scars because they were in the crease line under the breast. But I *still* never thought about it for me, until the next weekend when I was visiting some friends. A group of us were all sitting out on the patio, in the sunshine, and I said, 'Look at us, not one decent pair of tits between us.' And I told them about my client and her silicone implants. They were appalled. Every one of them said, ooh no, they'd never have *that* done, so I piped up, just to be different, 'Well, I would.' And that's how I made the decision, on the spur of the moment – it was a gesture of defiance really. Driving home that night I couldn't stop thinking about it, and I began to get very excited. The next morning I got up at the crack of dawn, rang my client to get the name of her plastic surgeon and made an appointment to see him.

'He asked me lots of questions about myself first. How did I feel about life, was I depressed, unhappy, had my marriage been happy? I had to convince him that everything was fine, I had a good social life, lots of friends, my business was going great guns, and I certainly wasn't planning to have it done in order to attract men. I'd divorced six years previously and had one serious relationship and plenty of boyfriends since; men had always said they liked my breasts. *I* was the problem. I was just fed up with being flat-chested.

'We discussed how big I wanted to go and I went back to see him with photographs. He told me that during the operation he always tried out two or three implants and there was always one that looked just right so in the end the final decision had to be left to him. He also warned me that I would be prone to encapsulation because I had very little breast tissue and he recommended that I have the more expensive polyurethane implants rather than the silicone ones.

'When I came round after the operation the nurse said to me, "You've got a beautiful pair of breasts" – as though I'd just given birth to twins! She lifted me up so I could have a look at them. They looked awful. I was wearing a sports bra and they were like two alien lumps sticking up. I left hospital that evening feeling as though I'd been run over by ten trucks. I was told to keep my bra on and imagine that I had my best dinner service under each arm – in other words I couldn't lift my arms up at all, just bend them from the elbow.

'My mum came to stay to look after me; I couldn't have managed without her. I couldn't even raise my arms to reach the work surface or fill the kettle for a cup of tea. After two days I went back to the surgery to have the dressing changed and the nurse took my bra off, and my breasts looked like rock-hard mountains. No one prepared me for how weird they would look at first. She remarked about some very bad bruising on my right hand side but neither of us thought any more about it. But when I got home I began to have this terrific pain where the bruising was and it travelled down my right arm too. It became unbearable.

'I asked my mother to ring the hospital and they got in touch with my surgeon who was operating in another hospital miles out of town. He rang back and told me it was probably a leaky blood vessel under the skin and could I get to him straight away so he could operate again to seal it off. My first thought was, Oh no, he's not going to take them out is he? I ended up getting a commuter train out of London on a Friday night before a bank holiday weekend, and having to stand in the aisle all the way with this enormous, painful throbbing breast. When I finally arrived he said he couldn't operate there and then because I'd had tea and biscuits a little while before, so I went into surgery first thing next morning.

'He couldn't replace the polyurethane implant once he'd taken it out because it's impossible to resterilise them properly, and as he didn't have another one with him he put a silicone implant in its place. He said he thought I'd prefer that to nothing at all. But after three months the silicone one started to go hard. I went back to the surgeon and he just squeezed it hard with his hand and it went off pop like a champagne cork and my breast just went all floppy again. Six weeks later it hardened again. I was pretty fed up by this time. My right bosom looked different, not so natural, so I had more surgery to replace the silicone implant with a polyurethane one. But over the past year this has hardened too – I'm thinking of having another one put in maybe in six months time.

'But no, despite all the hoo-ha I don't regret it at all. I consider it the best thing I've ever done in my life. I can grab anything now, put it on and feel

OK – even old T-shirts look good. I feel that now I'm as I should have been born, more of a woman.

'At first I wore tight, low-cut dresses all the time and enjoyed sashaying around at parties showing my new figure off, but I'm through that stage now. You can hardly see the scar on the left one because it's faded so much, but the scar under the right one is longer and thicker. But my boyfriends don't seem to notice. I didn't even tell the last one until we split up – and he'd had no idea.

'I've had more fun since I turned forty than ever before, and I think I look better too. I will have more plastic surgery, probably an eye-lift and collagen injections. I'm certainly not going to grow old gracefully – I'm going with a struggle!'

CASE HISTORY

Charlotte, forty, went on what can only be described as a plastic surgery binge, having under-eye bags removed, a nose job and collagen injections all in the space of six months. She runs a recruitment consultancy business with her husband and has two stepchildren.

'When I was twenty I vowed I would start putting money in my piggy bank so I could have a face-lift when I was forty. I was determined not to end up looking like an old bag. It's not that I'm vain; I don't really have any feeling for my looks at all, I don't know what I look like. As soon as I was old enough I grew my hair long, lightened it to blonde and started piling on the make-up to conform to an image that men wanted at that time. Now I'm stuck with it, I've got to keep it going, I can't suddenly change character, can I? And yet underneath I feel I'm really just a fat, little bumbly engineer like my father.

'My first husband was twenty years older than me so I always felt confident about my appearance, but my husband now is younger and he's so terrific I'd hate to lose him. I know that sounds ridiculous, why should we lose a man because of the way we look, but it does happen, doesn't it? And I have so many insecurities. About a year ago I started to look very tired and the children would say, oh Mummy you must have had a terrible day and it reminded me of the pity that I felt for my first husband's ex-wife. When I first met her she was about forty-four and although she was amazingly confident and had been very beautiful, now she looked so tired. A great rush of compassion welled up inside me and I thought, oh God, I never want another woman to feel like this about me. And of course in business it can so easily happen. The young women start to think of you as a mother figure and the men dismiss you as a silly old bag.

'I began by having the bags under my eyes removed so I wouldn't look so tired. I answered an advertisement for a cosmetic surgery clinic that I spotted in a glossy magazine. The operation was done under a local anaesthetic (with intravenous sedation) in a private hospital. I seemed to come to slightly when they were stitching me up but I wasn't really aware of it, I just saw darkness and flashing. I felt discomfort afterwards but no real pain. I was left with tremendous black eyes, but managed to get back to work after a week with the aid of dark glasses. I was so pleased with my eyes that I decided to have my nose fixed too.

'My nose seemed to have grown over the years. It had always been big but I began to notice that when I laughed a lot it threw a shadow across my upper lip. And when I got het up or excited it seemed to swell up and go red and start throbbing! The counsellor at the clinic suggested that I take a photograph of a nose I liked with me when I went to see the surgeon. I thought immediately of the actress Stephanie Powers, I've always liked her but I couldn't find any pictures so I took along some of another model with a lovely little nose. When the plaster came off (the most painful part of the whole thing by the way) I looked like Karl Malden! But now that the swelling has gone down I can see that actually he's done a very good job. He's given me a nose that fits my face. It's not that different to the old one, apart from being narrower and shorter. If it were just down to me I would probably go back and have a little bit more chopped off, but my husband thinks it's just fine so I probably won't bother.

'I told my PA what I was having done and I expect she told everybody in the office. The trouble with telling everybody is that they expect you to come back looking like someone out of *Dallas*, and of course you don't look that much different. But I think it's good to tell people. I think it's a great thing for equality. We can fight back. Ageing makes you very vulnerable as a woman. In business if you fight back by letting nature take its course it doesn't really work, because if you lose out because they think of you as a silly old thing, then you're not winning are you?

'It does seem to change some people's attitude to you. An old boyfriend of mine has suddenly started to take a great interest in me. I think he imagines that because I've had my face done I'm now up for a good time.

'The collagen injections have worked brilliantly too. It's probably been as good as having a face-lift. I've got lots of little lines on my forehead and around my mouth. I've always had jobs where I've had to concentrate a lot and stretch myself. So I've screwed up my face, worked overlong hours, drunk too much black coffee, worked in smoky atmospheres and now the wear and tear is showing. I did suffer a slight reaction to the injections though. My skin remained quite flushed and raised for at least a week afterwards.

'It's all been worth it because I look much healthier now. "You look *so* well," my mother keeps saying. Now when I get home after a hard day at the office, exhausted and ready to drop, the kids tell me I look radiant!'

CASE HISTORY

Helen, forty-seven, had a face- and eye-lift combined. She is a youth worker in an inner city area and is married with two teenage sons.

'I began the menopause at forty-two but didn't realise what was happening to me. For two years I suffered with terrible migraines and hot flushes. I was very short-tempered, put on weight and my face began to age dramatically. There were bags and lines under my eyes, the skin on my brow bone hung so far down that it touched my eyelashes, the lines around my mouth were sagging in folds. That was the worst part. Eventually I went to my doctor and he told me I was menopausal. But he gave me short shrift and offered no help.

'I didn't give up, I went back to the same practice but this time to a different doctor, one who had been my family doctor in the past. I explained the problem but only briefly because before I could finish he turned round and said to me, "Helen, you look about fifty-two." Well my whole world really crashed then. It was a major shock. But in the next breath he added, "It's not the end of the world, there's plenty we can do." He put me on Hormone Replacement Therapy and diuretic tablets and everything improved but my face. I still had the lines and the sagging skin from struggling along all those years without treatment. No matter what beauty treatment I tried, nothing worked. And I tried *everything*, one anti-ageing cream after another. I'd give them six weeks and then if there was no visible improvement I'd go on to another, more expensive one. I did facial exercises as well.

'In the end I saw an advertisement in a Sunday paper for cosmetic surgery. I decided to ring up and ask for information. And then I thought no, don't be so ridiculous, you can't possibly be thinking along these lines. So I just cut out the coupon and carried it around in my handbag for three months. Eventually this dog-eared coupon surfaced again and I thought, well, nothing has changed, I still look the same – let's go for it. I sent off for information and they sent back lots of literature and quoted prices and I made an appointment to see a counsellor. She was very helpful but much to my amazement looked very odd. From the chin up to the cheekbones she looked very good but her eyes and forehead were quite grotesque. The bags under her eyes were drooping on to her cheekbones. Apparently she was having her face lifted in stages and hadn't saved up enough for the top half yet!

'I decided to do some homework before making a commitment. I checked out the credentials of the surgeon and the anaesthetist in the *Medical Directory* and rang the council to make sure that the clinic where the operation would take place had been licensed by the health authority. Everything came up OK but I didn't want to rush into it. I went to my doctor to get his opinion and he virtually threw me out: he said, "You're getting old, you must accept it." I thought, well, to hell with this, and went to see my old family doctor again and he said, "What a wonderful idea, Helen." He thoroughly approved and what's more, rang up a surgeon in Harley Street and fixed an appointment for me straight away. Despite the fact that this surgeon dealt with film stars and TV people his prices weren't much above those quoted by the clinic. But I still didn't say yes. In the end a friend suggested I try a cosmetic surgery clinic also in London that she'd heard was very good and I said to my friend, who'd come along with me on every appointment so far, let's have a choice of three.

'I just felt it was a wonderful set-up from the word go. The nurse counselled me brilliantly – she was sympathetic and thorough and asked me about my past medical history in great detail. She quoted prices and asked if I would like to leave a deposit – for £650! I was stunned. I thought, oh my God, I don't have anything like that sort of money with me, and then my girlfriend looked at me and nodded yes and opened her purse and took out £1,000 in cash. She said, "I knew this was going to be the right one. Go for it – it's the best of the lot." I booked up there and then and arranged it to fit in with the school half term.

'I didn't tell the people at work. I didn't think it was anybody else's business and anyway a lot of young men work at the youth centre and I didn't think they'd understand. I told them I was having some eye operations.

'I gave up smoking the month before as advised. The operation took three and a half hours. As I was coming to I thought, okay, I'm going to get pain now, but I didn't, there was just a feeling of tightness, of being closed in very tight like a mummy. There were bandages around my head, a drain behind each ear and a drip in my arm. I didn't want to move my head or neck from side to side but I could blink and I could speak. I had lots of antibiotic cream in my eyes which made my vision blurred (at first I thought the op had affected my sight). I felt the odd twinge of discomfort but had some painkillers and managed to sleep beautifully through the night.

'The next morning I had a bath and looked at myself for the first time. At first I thought my face would never get better, but then once I'd got over the shock and looked more closely I was surprised at the lack of bruising. My face was so swollen I couldn't make out whether there was any improvement or not. A nurse washed my hair and I began to feel more human. My husband sent a car for me and wearing headscarf and dark glasses I was home by lunchtime.

'For the first two weeks I had to sleep in an upright position to prevent blood clots. This meant I ended up sleeping on the sofa downstairs! Three days later I had the stitches around my ears removed but I still had lots of "staples" in the back of my head which felt taut and uncomfortable and prevented me from turning my neck easily from side to side. They were removed a week later and to my horror I discovered there were about fifty of the things. When I stepped outside the clinic afterwards I was gripped by a terrific pain that ran from the crown of my head to the base of my neck. I felt sick, unstable and very ill. I took paracetamol, slept all afternoon and by the next day the pain had gone.

'My son, who works in catering, made up icepacks for me to place on my eyes and cheekbones and the sides of my face to reduce the swelling and some bruising which was beginning to come up on my cheeks. I used them for fifteen minutes, three times a day. Within two weeks I was able to go back to work.

'No one guessed I'd had a face-lift. One man who I've worked with for ten years told me I looked fabulous. "There's something different about you, Helen," he said, "but I can't work out what it is." Another male friend who did know about it told me it was a terrific improvement, "and so subtle". These kind of comments made it all worthwhile. I feel more confident, more feminine – at last my face reflects the way I feel inside.

'I can't believe that I've actually got *eyelids* again – I can wear eye make-up if I want to. Before there would have been nowhere to put it and it would just have looked awful if I'd tried. I've still got deep furrows between my nose and mouth – laughter lines really – but I've booked up for collagen injections to lessen these. I've changed my hair colour and I'm having my front teeth capped to finish the new look off. The whole thing has been such a boost to my morale.'

EIGHT

The Best Of Health and a Beautiful Body

'Loving your body is the best beauty treatment of all'

———————

'All women become like their mothers. That's their tragedy.
No man does. That's his.'
Oscar Wilde

———————

When we were twenty, we never listened to our mothers banging on about how we should take better care of ourselves, because the last thing we wanted was to turn out looking anything like them. But now, it seems, that sterling generation of no-nonsense matrons was right all along. These days bookshops and magazine racks groan with glossy, complicated diet and exercise advice, which, after close analysis, turns out to be just the same old stuff that our mothers tried to hammer into our brains when we were young. There are no magic cures and few new diseases – most health problems really can be put down to bad personal habits and paying attention to Mother's rules can sort them out. Thus eating your greens, an apple a day, going easy on the fat and sugar, getting plenty of fresh air and exercise, cutting out smoking and too much alcohol, staying out of the sun and getting plenty of sleep really *do* do more for you than all the diet supplements, therapies and exercise equipment that money can buy.

Of course when we were twenty we didn't *want* to look healthy the way we do now. In the sixties it was fashionable to be thin, pale, hollow-eyed and neurotic. If you could develop manic depression you were really happening, and to have tuberculosis put you right up there with the Pre-Raphaelite goddesses. We didn't *want* to be tanned, muscular, energetic and happy, man that was sooooo uncool. Anyone who *exercised* was regarded with the horror reserved for the old school gym mistress. Lying languidly on sofas smoking joints to Dylan's 'Desolation Row' or practising the lotus position to Ravi Shankar's sitar was as near to limbering up as we ever got, and a workout session meant trying to work out the meaning of the lyrics (generally filthy) on Mothers Of Invention records while our brains reeled with chemical substances. Food meant black coffee and cigarettes; Mars Bars and chip butties if we felt we really must put something in our concave stomachs. Although thin, we never felt emaciated enough, so diets of hard-boiled eggs, grapefruit and Ryvita were frequently embarked on.

Of course this couldn't go on, and round about twenty-five we started to discover food. Living with men, or even getting married, meant learning how to cook – and a whole new world opened up. After the austerity of the post-war decades, food was everywhere and fast food chains were born. Suddenly there were hamburgers, pizza, pasta, fifty-two varieties of ice-cream – temptations at every turn. And then there was TV. We stopped going out to all-night happenings and burning off five thousand calories a night – we stayed in, cooked dinners and watched the box. Before the seventies, there had been nothing but *The Man From Uncle, Ready Steady Go* and *Emergency Ward Ten* to watch. Now there was more happening on TV than there was outside. So the weight crept up, the physical activity stopped, but the smoking and drinking carried on apace.

It was inevitable that all this self-indulgence would catch up with us one day. In fact it's a miracle that some of our forty-year-old bodies haven't completely fallen apart.

Forty is definitely the right age for taking stock. Your twenty-year-old body may have disappeared along with your crushed velvet loons and mirrored waistcoat, but it's still buried in there somewhere trying to get out. The first step to recovery is to admit that Mother was always right, and that you're going to have to start living sensibly after all.

HOW A BODY AGES
(Or why you must accept looking older at forty than you did at twenty.)

No matter how well you've looked after yourself all these years, and no matter what you do to yourself now, you're never going to look twenty again. This doesn't mean you can't look as *good* as you did at twenty, and perhaps feel even better, but it's going to be a different way of looking and feeling good.

If you really get yourself together now and maintain all your good habits, you could still look forty when you're sixty. But the days of being naturally fit, however badly you abuse and neglect yourself, are *over*. From now on, everything you put in your body, and the amount you exercise it or not, *counts*.

There are certain facets of ageing you cannot change, many that you can. Just staying thin won't keep you looking young – dancers at forty may have bodies that look twenty but their faces keep abreast of the times. Plumper women often have faces with rounder, younger contours, but their bodies can look fifty or more. At forty, finding the balance is the key. It may well suit you better to carry a little more weight than you did at twenty, as fat distributes itself differently as you age.

FAT FACTS
An average woman of twenty has approximately 26 per cent body fat. By thirty this has gone up to 33 per cent, by forty to 35 per cent, and by fifty to 42 per cent. But this isn't irreversible – women who exercise vigorously over forty often show body fat ratios as low as 22 per cent, less than a twenty-year-old. Sedentary women who do not exercise show a classic weight gain of one pound a year between twenty and forty, and most of this fat goes to the hips and thighs. The only way to shift it is to eat less than you did at twenty-five.

As you age, muscle and bone density decreases, so the body needs fewer calories to fuel them up. Excess energy is stored in the fat cells. For every decade past twenty, your calorie requirements decline by 2 per cent, so a woman who ate 2,500 calories at twenty-five to maintain her weight will need just 2,250 at forty.

In adolescence, excess weight gets distributed around the body, but in your thirties and forties it accumulates on the hips and thighs. The female hormone oestrogen is mostly responsible for this. By your fifties and sixties it will go to your waistline. If you carry on gaining one pound a year, through not changing your diet and exercise habits, by sixty you'll be decidedly dumpy. The effects of gravity and poor posture will further exacerbate excess weight problems, making the body look droopy and saggy. Many

overweight and out-of-shape women over forty are inevitably showing the
results of decades of self-indulgence. For many women food takes the place
of more active interests. Food is seen as a demonstration of love, thus
women cook endless meals to nurture their families. And calorie-laden cakes
and sweets are taken regularly as 'treats' to fill up the gaps in our lives
caused by boredom, disappointment and frustration. Most fat people have
bad food habits. Breaking them is the key.

THE METABOLISM DEBATE

Do fat people have slower metabolisms? And if so, can they speed them up?

Obesity can only occur when there is an excess of energy intake over
expenditure, but this discrepancy may not arise simply because one person
is eating more than average. Doctors at the Medical Research Council's
Dunn Nutrition Unit in Cambridge have found new techniques for
measuring human energy intake and expenditure in an ultra-precise way.
Through studying babies during their first years of life, they have found that
although all the babies ate exactly the same amount, some put on more
weight than others, and these same overweight babies expended less energy
than the normal weight ones when they were awake. When asleep,
however, all the babies burned the same amount of energy. This suggests
that the ones who would become fat were less lively and moved around less
when awake than the normal weight ones. Generally, they were considered
to be more placid. So fatness in babies is not due to eating more than usual.

Similar studies have been carried out amongst a group of Pima Indians
living in Arizona. This tribe were chosen because they are known to be very
likely to put on weight – by their early twenties, 85 per cent of the Pima
population is obese. By keeping track of the Indians over a period of two
years, scientists found that the ones who gained the most weight were not
eating more, but burning fewer calories. It only amounted to eight calories
fewer a day burnt up than was normal for their body sizes, but that was
enough for them to gain nine pounds a year.

So it really could be that more relaxed people who generally move about
less, burn up less energy than their nervier friends, and so have a tendency
to plumpness all through their lives. Moreover, obesity tends to be inherited,
so plump, placid mothers have plump, placid babies.

In trials where both fat and thin people are overfed, both groups put on
weight at the same rate, so it seems that naturally thin people don't have
metabolisms that can cope with however much they eat. The person who
eats like a horse and never gains any weight is a myth.

It really does seem that the only way to take weight off and keep it off is to
eat less and move about more over quite a long period of time. Weight lost
quickly through very low calorie diets will always be regained because your
metabolism responds by slowing right down as your body is literally being
starved. When you lose weight fast you lose a disproportionate ratio of
muscle to fat. So although you would expect your metabolism to drop 5 per
cent for every 5 per cent of muscle tissue lost, it actually drops by double that

amount, as your body tries to conserve energy. However, as your weight stabilises, your metabolism returns to normal. So if you lose weight, you'll be able to maintain your new weight only by eating less than you did when you were heavier, permanently.

HOW MUCH DOES EXERCISE HELP TO KEEP WEIGHT DOWN?

Studies show that people who diet without exercising regain the weight far more quickly than those who exercise during dieting. Exercise seems to increase metabolism by 2 or 3 per cent over the next twenty-four hours, so the more you exercise, the longer you can keep your fat-burning revved up. An hour of exercise at a pitch intense enough to speed up your heart rate, three times a week, is enough to keep metabolism in top gear. (More about this in 'Finding Your Exercise Routine'.)

Of course the way you look is not the only reason for losing weight. Excess weight also contributes to the development of diabetes, high blood pressure, cardiovascular disease, breast cancer and arthritis. And a shapely body isn't the only reason to exercise – deconditioned muscles reveal under the microscope the atrophy of cells and a loss of contractability. Less flexible muscles are more susceptible to strains, pulls and cramping. Your heart is the most important muscle of all. Working your large muscle groups forces the heart to work harder in turn, keeping it strong and in peak condition.

So we're really sorry, and we'd like to tell you different, but there really is no way out of confrontation with your destiny. If you've managed to resist it so far, and you're not a total physical wreck, it just goes to show how much your body really is on your side. But you won't be able to put it off much longer, and most of us had to face it long ago. The leg-lift and the semi-skimmed milk are in your future. Accept it with good grace and you may well find the rewards more than repay the regrets.

TAKING MORE CARE OF YOURSELF

The time is right now. Just because you're not overweight, stiff-jointed or tired all the time doesn't mean you can avoid these annoyances indefinitely. Changing your lifestyle will not only lengthen your life, it will radically alter the quality of your life meanwhile.

There's nothing new scientifically, and it won't cost you any money. Taking more care of yourself simply means incorporating all the following habits into your daily lifestyle.

EATING A BALANCED DIET

Too much food hastens ageing – Dr Roy Walford in America has found that underfeeding rats doubles or even trebles their lifespan. He is currently experimenting on himself, so we'll have to wait over forty years to see if he's right about the effect of undernutrition on humans. However, it is generally accepted that too much fat, sugar and cholesterol ages cells whereas anti-oxidants such as vitamins C and E can retard ageing at cellular level. This means:

✸ *Eat less* white flour, salt, red meat, sugar, animal fats.

✸ *Eat more* vegetables, fruits, grains, low-fat milk and water.

✸ *Take regular exercise.* The benefits are the same whether you are twenty-five or sixty-five. Exercising at the right intensity can give you a 20 per cent improvement in muscle strength, and up to 25 per cent improvement in your maximum oxygen intake, taking twenty years off your calendar age. But exercise must be careful to avoid damage to muscles, so adequate warming up and cooling down exercises are essential.

✸ *Stop smoking.* Apart from contributing to various cancers and heart disease, it causes digestive problems and ruins your skin.

✸ *Cut down on alcohol:* 14 units a week is your safe limit. One unit equals a half pint of beer, a glass of wine, a measure of spirits or a small sherry. Over 25 units a week will damage your health.

✸ *Protect your skin from the sun.* The days of tanning are gone for you. The sun can give you cancer, and at the very least badly ages your skin.

✸ *Examine your breasts regularly* and report any differences at once to your doctor.

✸ *Have regular smears* Demand one every three years on the National Health, and if you can afford to go privately have them yearly.

✸ *Have regular blood pressure checks:* it shouldn't go higher than 140/90.

✸ *Give up the pill* – you should have done so at thirty-five.

✸ *Investigate hormone replacement therapy* if you're entering early menopause.

✸ *Take calcium supplements* to ward off brittle bones later.

✸ *Take vitamin and mineral supplements* if there is some reason why you can't eat a wide range of foods.

✸ *Look after your teeth* and floss regularly.

✸ *Avoid excess stress.* Find relaxation techniques to suit you.

❋ *Investigate alternative therapies* that may cure problems conventional medicine cannot.

MAKE PEACE WITH YOUR BODY TYPE

Getting a positive body image is about the most favourable thing you can do for yourself – a bad body image is a constant drain on your energy, self-esteem and enjoyment of sex. For many women, their entire social life can be controlled by an obsession with their weight. Most of us have terribly unrealistic expectations of how our bodies should be. The current ideal is ultra slender with big boobs – a well-nigh impossible combination without surgical intervention. And the women who have this miraculous body weight arrangement are not actually more desired than flat-chested, big-bottomed ones. Men really don't care half as much about our figures as we do. Just as many men shy away from big bosoms and love ample bottoms as go for the model-girl type.

Our obsessions with our bodies are not really about men. If you feel bad about your body it's because you feel bad about yourself. Women blame their bodies for everything else that is wrong in their lives.

At forty it is time to make friends with your body. It's stuck around this long, despite all the abuse you've heaped upon it, so don't you think it's time to accept it and give it some love? Most of us could do with some attention to diet and exercise, but we should do it to pamper our bodies and to feel healthy, not with an obsessive sense of self-denial and self-disgust.

True, men often are extremely rude about women's bodies, as if they have a right to comment on every passing form. Usually the more imperfect the man, the more he is contemptuous of physical 'flaws' in women. These men are sexually inadequate, and are passing on their low self-images to the women they are close to. If you live with a man who wishes you had bigger boobs or a smaller bum, ask him why he wishes you were different. Forty is an age where women often rush out for breast implants or liposuction in order to save their marriage or attract new men – but it's their partners who need changing, not their bodies.

By all means work on your body to get it into its most fit and attractive state – but only do so from a position of loving your fundamental shape the way it is. If you are short and curvy or tall and willowy, you will still be that way after all the diet and exercise routines in the world – but you'll be the best your body type can be.

All types of figures have been fashionable at one time or another; women who are tall and slim just happen to be lucky right now. Emma Hamilton had Lord Nelson in a constant lather when she was fourteen stone, and Rubens and Renoir would never have wanted to paint Victoria Principal, deeming her quite deformed.

Elizabeth Taylor is a sexy woman fat or thin, but she just can't come to terms with herself. Jane Fonda would probably look more appealing if she stopped the diet, exercise and plastic surgery altogether, and Sophia Loren has always been the most universally fancied star, while making an hourglass look like a cricket stump.

Ignore, too, all that stuff about ectomorphs, endomorphs and mesomorphs. Most of us are slim in some places and plump in others, and defy categorisation.

Decide *your* type is the *best* type, and then set about dressing to show off what you've got. Everyone else perceives you as exactly as attractive as you perceive yourself. You owe yourself good health – but most of all you owe yourself self-respect.

GETTING THE MOTIVATION TO CHANGE

To be conscious of your body and to take care of it well increases your well-being and self-esteem. To feel your body has slipped out of your control makes your whole personality suffer.

If you're more overweight than is good for you, and you can't bring yourself to exercise, you must examine what's holding you back. It's far more likely to be complex psychological problems than the fact that you are greedy, lazy and undisciplined. Many people who have no control over their weight are paragons of self-control in *every* other aspect of their lives. The weight is the one area where they allow themselves to be weak. It's as if it is a rebellion against having to be perfect right down the line.

We believe there are different sorts of fat people. There are the *fated fat*, who tend to be placid, nurturing and open-hearted. They are generous with everything else as well as food – they hate to do anything in half measures and they are over-abundant in personality and emotional strength. Claire Rayner, Sheila Kitzinger and Nancy Roberts are all examples of these, and it really wouldn't suit them to lose weight at all. Interestingly, all these women are happily and longstandingly married, unlike many of their svelter colleagues.

Secondly there are the *fearful fat*. These eat to assuage anxiety and stress. Instead of the fight or flight response when confronted with danger, they eat. Sweet sugary snacks temporarily sedate their neuroses but it's a vicious circle of stress and self-hatred. If you are a fearful fat person, you must first find another way of dealing with anxiety, *then* you can diet. Take away your starchy crutches before you're ready, and depression and self-pity quickly set in. For you, exercise, relaxation techniques and finding a less stressful lifestyle should come before trying to diet.

Thirdly there are the *frustrated fat*. A lot of inner rage and disappointment percolates in the breast of the frustrated fat. Families who take you for granted, lack of career direction and hostility towards men can turn the slenderest maiden into one of these. Again, to find the motivation to get fit, you'll have to put the rest of your life in order first.

Just tackling the diet and exercise issue without confronting why you overate in the first place leaves none of the inner conflicts resolved, and eating disorders can follow. Anorexia and bulimia are very common amongst fortysomethings who can't face the desert within, and trying to control their bodies is just side-stepping the issue of getting some control over their lives.

The motivation to change twenty years of bad habits must come from the realisation that your body has got nothing to do with the other problems in your life. Being slim and attractive won't solve your money problems, your fears for your children or the fact that your husband is having an affair, but it will boost your self-esteem and show the world how highly you value yourself. You really have to love yourself the best – others always take you at your own self-evaluation.

Fit people are more assertive, more in control of their lives, more at peace with themselves. Next time you have a negative experience, don't reach for food. Nurture your body with some loving care instead. The stronger you feel, the more you'll be able to deal with life's endless parade of problems.

Pamper your body instead of punishing it, and it'll become your closest ally in helping you get exactly where you want to be.

HOW TO DIET

To diet may well be the most difficult thing you've ever had to do in your life. To those of us who are not over-fond of resisting temptation, having to refuse the opportunity for some oral gratification is like asking a baby not to suck. Perhaps eating has always been a way of warding off anxiety – when our ancient ancestors knew hard times were ahead and there was no telling where the next meal might come from, they stuffed themselves to capacity at every opportunity. Although it's very unusual to go hungry in the Western world, we still subconsciously feel this need to stay as full as possible all the time, to give us a sense of security.

You can't diet successfully until you accept that this unconscious insecurity has got to be dispelled another way. Food won't keep you safe – it just temporarily sedates you. You are in a vicious circle that you have to break. If you were fit and lean, you would feel stronger and more able to cope with anxiety, but to get fit and lean you need to get rid of the anxiety that stops you dieting in the first place.

Some people are jolted into breaking the vicious circle by a painful event – a rejection, an insult, a total humiliation. You read stories in *Slimming* magazine of women who suddenly shed six stone in six months after being fat for years, as the result of hearing this click in their heads when they saw some particularly horrible holiday snap, or overheard some grisly remark. In a way, the more overweight you are to begin with, the easier it is to start dieting, as you know it could be your weight or your life. But if you only have two or three stone to lose – not enough so that you look terrible, but enough for you to loathe yourself undressed – then you need a stronger incentive to start.

WOMEN AND FOOD

The brain stimuli associated with anxiety and hunger are very similar, so it's no surprise that women mistake the former for the latter. Deep-seated anxieties stemming from incidents way back in early childhood can still be hanging over your life in your forties. It's not enough to dismiss fat people as greedy – given the choice most of them would rather have a slim body than a lifetime of pigging out, but food really is the fat woman's drug. Sweet things particularly remind us of the security we felt on our mothers' knees.

Before marriage, even the most anxious women manage to keep their weight down through stringent dieting – *then* we had the time and energy to devote to disciplining ourselves. But with marriage and children comes an environment that can seem totally centred around food. If your marriage is happy and you feel loved, you can gain weight rapidly because you're constantly shopping and cooking up loving feasts for your dear ones. If your marriage is unhappy, weight soars even higher as snacks fill up the hours of loneliness, boredom and lack of sex. Some husbands like to keep their wives fat and depressed because it suits them to have a captive housekeeper who's too demoralised to run off with the milkman.

Many modern women have a complex and tortured relationship with food. In our society to be slim means to be successful and sexually attractive – a competitor. To be fat means to opt out of the rat race, but also to feel guilty and self-doubting.

To diet successfully you must want to be slim and join the participators, rather than to eat doughnuts at home. If you are fat now, you must ask yourself, 'Why don't I really want to lose weight?'

Do you associate slimness with sexuality? Are you afraid that if you lose weight you'll leave your husband because he doesn't satisfy you? Or that you'll feel so energetic you'll never be able to put up with being cooped up at home? Are you afraid that you'll want to start putting yourself first for a change?

What women must do is to dissociate slimness from other issues. Slimness is not about being more loved, sexy, successful, popular, rich. It is first and foremost a *health issue*, and this is the only way to approach it.

At forty, you've got to get fit in order to live the next forty years healthily and happily. And at forty you've got to finally face up to and banish those inner fears that hold you back. Make peace with your past and make peace with your body. Treat it well so that it will serve you better, not because you see it as the means to success in the outside world. Dieting should not be seen as a battle, but as a means of caring for yourself. Not self-denial, but self-nurture. Although a diet has to be permanent in the sense that you will have to change your eating habits for life, you can still eat all your favourite things in the future – just not every day, and not indiscriminately. Chocolates, cream cakes, pasta, pizza and curries are all out there waiting for you. It's how you eat every day that is important – you need a basic eating plan that doesn't include these things, so as to balance the days when you just have to binge. Sticking to a daily diet is not so difficult when you know the rules and have made a pact with yourself to obey them. If you can trust yourself to eat sensibly most of the time, then the occasional calorie bomb is not going to blow apart your entire slimming plan.

DIET RULES

Make food less important in your life. Love your body more than you love eating. If you have problems with life's stresses, seek another way to cure yourself of anxiety. Many people lose weight during psychoanalysis. Food is for nourishment, not to drug you.

Find alternatives to eating. If food has become your primary source of enjoyment and relaxation, develop other interests. Every time you have a desire to eat, do something else instead.

Don't combine eating with other activities. When you eat, really concentrate on the food. Don't watch TV, talk on the phone or read at the same time. Otherwise every time you do any of the above it will act like a trigger making you want to eat.

Tolerate hunger. If you are so afraid of being hungry that you make sure you never experience it, you can find yourself constantly munching. Stop eating between meals so that your appetite has time to regain its normal function.

Be aware of your dependence on oral gratification. On a bad day, you can feel like you consist of just a mouth and a stomach. Food is meant to give you energy, like putting fuel in a car, not to fill up an emotional void. When it's mouth hunger rather than stomach hunger that you feel, chew gum, eat fruit or drink herbal tea or water.

Don't tell anybody you're dieting. Just say you're trying to eat more healthily. If you say you're dieting and people see you eating chocolate, they can't resist commenting, even though *you* know the chocolate is a treat you've worked towards for days before.

Don't crash diet. The benefits will be very temporary. It's okay for a week or two before a holiday or a special party, but be aware that you will regain all the weight when you return to normal eating. Long-term crash dieting is positively bad for you as you will burn muscle protein as well as fat stores, and your metabolism will slow right down triggering the body into survival mode.

Eat regular meals. Three balanced meals a day is still the best way to diet. If you need snacks in between, choose fresh fruit and vegetables, or a savoury like Marmite on Ryvita. You must break the habit of turning to biscuits and sweets to bridge that gap.

When you must have chocolate buy one small bar. Never store it at home or buy the family-size pack.

Substitute low calorie alternatives. For cream use yoghourt, tofu or fromage blanc. For sugar use artificial sweeteners (though it's better to try to educate your tastebuds away from sweet foods). For sauces use vegetable stock, herbs and cream substitutes. When frying use a non-stick pan and an oil spray. For salt, use garlic and herbs.

Eat more fibre. Wholegrain breads and cereals, biscuits, fruit and vegetables are all filling and good for the bowels.

Make sure you get adequate calcium and potassium: skim or low fat milk, cheese, more fruit and vegetables.

Work on your body image. Believe you can be slim, and constantly picture yourself that way. Imagine how you will feel, especially your lovely flat stomach. The overweight person usually has a fat self-image, and your appetite centre works through the subconscious to keep you that way. Think of yourself as slim, and your appetite obliges by wanting less food to make you that way.

Set goals you can achieve. Accept that you won't lose more than two pounds a week. You could lose ten pounds in two weeks if you went on a very low calorie diet, but you won't be able to maintain this. It may be a good idea to start off a diet this way to give you motivation, but be prepared to regain some weight even when you go on to 1,500 calories a day.

BE PREPARED TO CARRY ON DIETING THROUGH THE 'PLATEAU' PERIOD

In the first few days of dieting, the main weight loss is caused by water, not fat loss. The body's natural reaction thereafter is to retain fluid. The rate of fat loss continues, but the weight loss can be obscured by this fluid retention. Understand what is happening and persevere, then this excess fluid will eventually be excreted by the kidneys. Whenever you binge in the middle of a diet, a really massive fluid gain can occur – causing five pounds weight gain in a day. Don't take diuretics, just continue your diet, and your weight loss will stabilise again.

DEVISE YOUR OWN DIET

We've purposefully not given a set diet here, because every person has her own individual way of restricting food. You don't need to be told about calorie counts or which are the 'good' and 'bad' foods, because unless you've been on an interplanetary cruise for the last twenty years, you can hardly have failed to absorb all this information through the press and TV. Set meal plans are a waste of time – who knows what you're going to fancy eating Wednesday lunchtime? It could well *not* be stir-fried endive and cottage cheese. Some days can be a cheese day, some days a rice day, another day you've just got to have chicken. The way to stay in touch with your appetite and tastebuds is to decide on a daily basis what you're going to eat. Before a period you may well crave carbohydrates more than at any other time in the month. Days when you're desperate for chocolate you could plan a chocolate lunch. Suiting youself is the key, then you won't feel deprived and brow-beaten by some Nazi eating regime that you hate by day three. Of course it is useful to keep your daily food allowance between 1,000 and 1,500 calories, so a good calorie counter is essential.

DIET SABOTEURS AND SAVIOURS
Addictions
The most common food cravings are for sugar, chocolate and caffeine.

Sugar
The craving for a high sugar snack is usually the result of low blood sugar. When the blood glucose falls, we experience a low, characterised by fatigue and an inability to concentrate. A sugary snack sends blood sugar soaring, and in order to get the levels under control again the pancreas produces large quantities of insulin. The abundance of insulin causes the blood sugar levels to plummet again, leaving you craving for yet another sweet treat. To ensure a steady supply of sugar to the blood and keep levels constant, eat plenty of complex carbohydrates. This means wholegrain bread, brown rice, rolled oats, potatoes, chick peas and lentils. Beware of too much sugar in dried fruit, honey and fruit juice. Deficiencies of magnesium, chromium, vitamin B6, potassium and zinc aggravate low blood sugar problems, so you may want to take a balanced vitamin and mineral supplement.

Taking regular exercise keeps blood sugar steady.

Before your period you may well crave sweets more than normally, as your metabolic rate increases in the last two weeks of your cycle and progesterone, which stimulates the appetite, increases. Regular complex carbohydrate snacks should keep this under control. Doctors now claim that sugar is so bad for you that it should carry a government health warning, like tobacco. Use sugar for special treats only, never sprinkled on cereal or in coffee and tea.

Chocolate
This is Maggi's particular failing and it's very hard to substitute with anything else. Nothing tastes quite like chocolate. It contains the stimulants theobromine and theophylline, also phenylethylamine which is a chemical we produce naturally when feeling sexually attracted. No wonder He goes to all that trouble just because the lady likes Milk Tray. Actually anyone who likes Milk Tray is not a true chocaholic – the hardliners like it dark, strong and unadulterated by gooey centres.

Substituting carob bars or opting for low-calorie chocolate drinks doesn't work when you crave the real thing. Even Death By Chocolate can turn out to be a charlatan. We suggest you buy the smallest, darkest, richest bar you can find, and eat it very, very slowly. To do this once or even twice a week won't sabotage your diet, but you must see chocolate for what it is: a satanic plot to keep you enslaved and unable to achieve thirty-six inch hips. Take control of it before it conquers you.

Caffeine

This stimulant is found in coffee, tea, cola, chocolate and many over-the-counter drugs. Caffeine is very addictive. Four cups of tea or coffee a day is okay; one or two cups can be positively good for you, stimulating the central nervous system and the secretion of stomach acid and urine, and possibly increasing the amount of fat burned for energy. Doctors now say it may speed up the basal metabolic rate by about 10 per cent. The traditional cup of coffee after dinner may actually help you digest a heavy meal.

If you are consuming too much caffeine, cutting down can lead to the extreme withdrawal symptoms of headaches, irritability and lethargy. Wean yourself off slowly by consuming one cup less a day, substituting decaffeinated tea or coffee, or mineral water. Don't drink caffeine after eight o'clock in the evening as it will impair your sleep.

Food allergies

Allergies to certain foods or chemicals can aggravate or even cause such conditions as asthma, hay fever, eczema, catarrh, sinusitis and tonsillitis. Common allergens are milk products, wheat, food colourings, flavourings and preservatives.

If you suffer from constant exhaustion, irritability, indigestion and bowel disorders, a sensitivity to certain foods could be the reason. The most usual way nutritionists discover which foods create allergic reactions is by excluding the most common allergens from the diet. First dairy produce will be removed, then grains. In a few cases, it may also be necessary to remove eggs, meat and fish. In addition, foods containing monosodium glutamate should be avoided. After a few weeks, foods are gradually reintroduced. An immediate reaction will occur when the danger food is eaten. Bit by bit the boundaries of which foods are acceptable and which are not can be defined.

Stone Age people ate little dairy produce and grew no grains, so these foods are relatively new to the human organism. It's little wonder that some people cannot tolerate them.

Anti-oxidants

These are our defence against too many free radicals in the body, which interact with cells and can either destroy them or affect their structure so they reproduce incorrectly. Free radical production is strongly promoted by cigarette smoking, and diminished by adequate supplies of the anti-oxidant vitamins E and C from fresh fruit and vegetables. Further protection may come from mono-unsaturated fats, such as olive oil. It was thought at one time that polyunsaturates reduced cholesterol, but now researchers in Cambridge say that in processing polyunsaturates the body is more likely to generate free radicals. The mineral selenium is also thought to break down free radicals.

Cholesterol

A significant proportion of the brain is cholesterol, your nerves can't function without it, blood vessels produce it to provide lubrication, and sex hormones are made from it. At least half your cholesterol supplies are made in the liver, but you also get it from food. The higher your intake of saturated fat, the more cholesterol you make. If you have too much cholesterol in your system, lipoproteins in your blood carry it to dumping grounds on your artery walls, and the resultant clogging can lead to coronary heart disease. Five millimoles cholesterol per litre of blood is considered safe, six is bad and eight is dangerous.

Getting down to your ideal weight produces a fall in blood cholesterol levels, as does giving up smoking and taking more exercise. Animal fats are rich in cholesterol, so you should go easy on eggs, milk, cheese, butter, red meats and meat products. Some types of water-soluble dietary fibre can reduce blood cholesterol, so oats and beans are particularly helpful. Baked beans, kidney, flageolet and broad beans, and oat products such as porridge and oat bran muffins can all decrease blood cholesterol. Include a serving of one every day.

Fish oils containing omega-3 fatty acids also reduce cholesterol levels. Salmon and mackerel are particularly high in omega-3.

There's no need to panic too much about cholesterol, though, because women have built-in defences against the storage of fatty deposits in their arteries that men don't have. Women don't suffer much risk of heart disease before they're fifty. After the menopause cholesterol seems to accumulate more rapidly. By sixty, rates of heart disease among men and women are about equal.

DETOXIFYING DIETS

The closer to nature the food you eat, the healthier you'll be, but in these days of high pressure lifestyles it's difficult to find time to shop for and prepare unadulterated food. The resultant intake of chemicals through processed foods, and too much fat and sugar through eating high-taste low-nutrition snacks can lead to an accumulation of toxins in the digestive tract, leaving you feeling tired, bloated, nauseous, spotty and prone to headaches.

A detoxifying diet eliminates poisons from the body through the kidneys, lungs, bowels and skin. The programmes are usually ten days in length, and though you'll feel like hell while you're going through it, you should end up feeling good as new at the end. Some detox gurus swear that this is the only way to get rid of cellulite as well, deeming this bumpy fat to be the result of your body choosing a place far from vital organs – your thighs – to dump toxic waste. This has not been proven, but it's worth a try if normal dieting has failed to shift this unsightly fat.

A ten day detoxifying diet is very, very stringent, and it's likely that you won't feel at all well as your body experiences withdrawal symptoms from all your normal foods. Caffeine withdrawal can be particularly marked. But it really does form a brilliant launching pad to set you off on a lifetime of reformed eating, knowing that your digestive system is clean and clear, ready to adapt to a healthier diet.

TEN DAY DETOX PLAN
Days one and two
Drink only bottled water (not tap water as this contains chemicals).

Days three to eight

Breakfast: two or three pieces of fruit, such as apples, pears, grapes, peaches, mangoes, melon, strawberries, raspberries, orange, grapefruit (avoid bananas). Make a fruit salad from a combination of these if you prefer. Plus: herbal tea with up to one teaspoon of honey.

Lunch and evening
Mixed salad of any vegetables except potato
or mixed stir-fried vegetables
or steamed vegetables
Plus: one baked potato
or a cupful of brown rice
or two bananas
or one avocado
or two ounces of mixed unsalted nuts or seeds.
Flavour with small amount of olive oil and lemon juice.

Days nine and ten
As before, only add two slices of wholemeal bread a day, four ounces of live yoghourt and three ounces of fish or chicken, or two eggs cooked any way, or a bowl of lentil or bean soup. Finish with fresh fruit. Drink as much mineral water and herb tea as you want throughout the diet.

❀ No alcohol, no cigarettes, and no caffeine.

FRUIT FOR FITNESS
Most fruits have a very high vitamin and mineral content. They are rich in fibre, and due to their enzyme content, they are believed to trigger beneficial chemical reactions within the body. Some doctors these days believe that a high fruit diet can help prevent illness, rejuvenate the body and control diseases such as cancer. In foreign cultures where cancer is unknown, fruit usually features highly as a diet staple. The Pueblo Indians of New Mexico are said to reduce the risk of cancer by drinking a brew made from well-roasted kernels of cherries, peaches and apricots. American researchers have found that apricot kernels contain a substance they have called B-17

which may inhibit cancer growth, along with Carotene, found in apricots, peaches, prunes and mangoes.

Fructose in fruit is nearly 30 per cent sweeter than sucrose, so you need to use far less of it. Furthermore, fructose is absorbed much more slowly by the body and produces a more sustained supply of energy, so blood glucose levels stay more stable.

In other words, your body really does love fruit. If you're not used to eating much it can be difficult to change to a high fruit diet overnight – when you crave carbohydrates fruit seems too watery and acidic. Build up your consumption slowly: an apple a day at first, then two more pieces of fruit a day when you've adjusted to it. An all-day fruit fast is your next step, especially good after a heavy-calorie weekend, working up to three day fruit detox fasts to really spring-clean a sluggish digestion.

Try to develop the habit of snacking on fruit instead of sweets and biscuits, and money is much better spent on fruit than on vitamin supplements, because fruit gives you the fibre and minerals that pills can't offer.

THE NEW SLIMMING PILLS

Various drugs that speed up the metabolism are undergoing rigorous tests to see if they are safe enough for doctors to prescribe to the overweight. Researchers at Queen Elizabeth College are experimenting with a pill that contains Bromocriptine, a drug prescribed to women after childbirth to stop milk production. Researchers tried the pill on themselves and suffered no side-effects. Team leader Mr Derek Miller claims it speeded up the metabolic rate by 25 per cent. Exhaustive tests will be needed for several years to come before the drug can be put on the market, but two seventeen stone volunteers who tried it lost three stone each in eighteen weeks.

Another possibility is a mixture of aspirin and ephedrine, a drug found in some cough medicines. According to scientists at King's College, London, this combination can increase metabolism by as much as 50 per cent. A dose of one aspirin and six teaspoons of cough medicine containing ephedrine does the trick – the ephedrine makes you burn the calories while the aspirin prevents the ephedrine breaking down in the body before it can take effect. However, ephedrine is a stimulant and could be dangerous, especially to those with diabetes, the pregnant or those over sixty. Dieters should always consult their GPs before trying it as it may strain the heart.

Increasing metabolism artificially is unlikely ever to be as safe as doing the same through stepping up exercise.

VEGETARIANISM

More and more people are turning to a non-meat diet, for both health and humanitarian reasons. The horrors of battery farming and slaughterhouses are incentive enough, but the health angle is certainly persuasive. Vegetarians tend to have lower blood cholesterol, lower blood pressure, less risk of colon cancer, diabetes, appendicitis, piles and varicose veins.

Vegetarians are rarely obese, and tend to have stronger bones. There is a misconception among many people that a vegetarian diet is lacking in certain nutrients, and the anaemic vegetarian is a myth. Plenty of protein can be acquired from soya beans, wholemeal bread, nuts, pulses, milk, cheese and potatoes. Iron is plentiful in baked beans, wholemeal bread, pulses, nuts, dried fruit, leafy greens and brewer's yeast, and vitamin B12, a common deficiency in vegans, can be found in milk, soya protein, cheese and yeast extract. To be on the safe side, vegans, who don't eat dairy products, should take a B12 supplement, and also calcium.

VITAMIN AND MINERAL SUPPLEMENTS

A balanced diet provides all the nutrients most people need, and many doctors consider megadoses of vitamins and minerals a dangerous concept. The only supplements universally agreed to be useful are extra vitamin C for smokers, and the vitamin B complex for alcoholics. Excessive amounts of vitamins A and D are particularly dangerous.

In most countries, the government produces guidelines on the standard amount of vitamins required by the average person. Few minerals have recommended daily amounts (RDAs) in the UK, so we have to be guided by the American charts.

The term 'vitamin' covers a wide range of organic substances, all of which are essential to keep the body functioning, and all of which are available from food. If your diet is well balanced, i.e. you eat a wide range of natural unprocessed foods, then your vitamin intake should fulfil all your needs. However, if you eat a lot of carbohydrate and processed foods, you smoke and drink heavily and frequently take drugs, medicinal or otherwise, you may need more of certain vitamins. In these circumstances excess vitamins should be taken only under medical supervision. Fat-soluble vitamins A and D can build up to toxic levels when stored in the body, whereas excess water-soluble vitamins B and C usually pass out in the urine. Even so, too much of these can also cause problems.

In normal circumstances, only the very young, the elderly, and pregnant and breast-feeding women are ever likely to need extra vitamins, and pregnant women should not take vitamin A.

RECOMMENDED DAILY AMOUNTS OF VITAMINS

VITAMIN	RDA	FOOD SOURCE
A	750 micrograms	liver (100g-19,900mcg)
		carrots (100g-2,000mcg)
		spinach (100g-1,000mcg)
		cheese (75g-270mcg)
		milk, eggs, root vegetables, apricots
B1 (thiamin)	1mg	pork (100g-0.57 mg)
		wholemeal bread (100g-0.37mg)
		potatoes, brown rice, pulses
B2 (riboflavin)	1.3mg	liver (100g-4.4mg)
		cheese (75g-0.38mg)

VITAMIN	RDA	FOOD SOURCE
		milk (100g-0.17mg)
		cereal, wholemeal bread
B3 (niacin)	15mg	chicken (100g-5.9mg)
		cereals (30g-5mg)
		lean meat, liver, beans, pulses
B6 (pyridoxine)	2.2mg	wheatgerm (100g-95mg)
		bananas (100g-0.51mg)
		turkey (100g-0.44mg)
		yeast, liver, eggs, whole grains
B12	3 mcg	liver (100g-54mcg)
		white fish (100g-2mcg)
		eggs, milk, yeast
C	30mg	blackcurrants (50g-100mg)
		oranges (100g-50mg)
		grapefruit (75g-30mg)
		green pepper (50g-50mg)
		citrus fruits, leafy vegetables
D	unlimited, from sunlight	eggs, oily fish, margarine, fortified milk
E	unlimited	vegetable oils, milk, eggs, nuts, seeds
K	no RDA	leafy green vegetables, turnips, cereals

MINERALS

A wide range of minerals is also essential for good health, and slight deficiencies occur more easily than with vitamins. There are two groups of minerals: bulk minerals, required in substantial amounts in the diet, and trace minerals, required in only tiny amounts of less than 100mg a day. Minerals rarely exist on their own but combine with other elements. The balance is important. The mineral content of foods can be seriously impaired by refining and cooking – green vegetables can lose over half their potassium, magnesium and phosphorus, and a third of their zinc, calcium and iron when boiled in water. Vegetables should always be steamed. Mineral requirements increase during pregnancy and when breast-feeding, and when recovering from illness. Use of diuretics and high consumption of tea, coffee and alcohol can lead to the loss of potassium, magnesium and zinc.

USA RECOMMENDED DAILY AMOUNTS OF MINERALS

MINERAL	RDA	FOOD SOURCE
CALCIUM	800mg	milk (1 pint-700mg)
		cheese (100g-800mg)
		leafy vegetables, nuts. seeds, beans
IODINE	150mcg	fish and seafood, eggs, peanuts, cereals
IRON	18mg	liver, kidney, eggs, molasses
MAGNESIUM	300mg	green vegetables, eggs, milk, bread, peanuts
PHOSPHORUS	800mg	whole grains, vegetables, dairy products
ZINC	15mg	meat, nuts, eggs, wholewheat, rye, oats, milk, carrots

Selenium has been suggested to help protect tissues from wear and tear, some cancers and the effects of the ageing process. It should be taken with vitamin E, and is available in wholegrains, seafood and offal.

FINDING YOUR EXERCISE ROUTINE

The best reason for exercising I've ever heard comes from Debbie Moore of Pineapple. She says, 'The more you do, the more you can get away with indulging in all the things that made you unfit in the first place.' It's also true that exercise keeps ageing at bay more than *anything* else.

Many of us fantasise about exercising and achieving perfect thighs, but we also have a huge psychological block about even starting. The more stressed and riddled with low self-esteem you are, the more overweight and unfit, the less you want to confront how out of shape you have become. It's got nothing to do with being too busy or too lazy – you don't work out because you can't face any kind of confrontation with your body at all. We put off starting an exercise routine until we're settled, until we've dieted off some weight first, until we've moved house, started a new job, etc., etc.

There will never be any time better than the present. Exercise should be the fundamental thing that you do *before* anything else. It really can be the key to solving many if not all the other problems in your life.

Being fit not only develops you physically, it improves you mentally and spiritually too. It's very self-loving, an expression of high self-esteem. To be fully in touch with your body makes you much more self-accepting, self-reliant and complete.

Many women avoid exercise because they hate their bodies and want to ignore them. The further your body has slipped out of your control, the further away the possibility of fitness seems. Images of lean aggressive people competing at gyms and aerobic classes put off the gentler, more introverted souls. But your own personal exercise plan doesn't have to involve you in any of this showy stuff. You can start quietly and gently, and build up very, very slowly.

Exercise for you should be a holistic activity – relaxing tension, strengthening your body and clarifying your mind.

At forty, your body still has the capacity to become slender, graceful and strong. At no age does muscle become incapable of increasing in capacity, and at forty you can still regain your twenty-five-year-old shape. And you can do it in a matter of months.

Many women don't give attention to their bodies because they are so busy catering for everyone else's needs, they don't feel able to contemplate *one more thing*. We neglect ourselves almost on purpose, as if we feel we don't deserve to 'waste' time attending to ourselves. But if you're fit, everything else in your life becomes easier to handle. Putting aside two to three hours a week to spend on your body doesn't seem too much to ask of even the busiest individual. All you've got to decide is when to do it, and what kind of exercise you want to do.

HOW TO CHOOSE

The minimum amount of exercise you need to do to get results is three half-hour sessions a week. For all-round fitness you need to choose exercise methods that provide all three of the following factors:

* Flexibility
* Strength
* Aerobic Fitness.

FLEXIBILITY

This type of exercise increases joint mobility and strengthens the surrounding muscles, thus improving posture and warding off arthritis. A supple, relaxed body comes from stretching the muscles rather than building bulk. Systems such as Medau, Pilates and Feldenkrais work on flexibility, as do yoga and dance. Choose one class a week from these.

Yoga

Yoga is a particularly holistic flexibility system. This ancient classical philosophy believes that the mind, body and soul are one, and should always be in harmony. Emphasis is placed on body alignment and breathing, so it is an excellent way to combat the effects of ageing. As you get better at it you'll find your body doing things you never dreamt possible. Beginners use ten to thirty positions which work all the muscle groups. Yoga also builds strength, so combined with an aerobic exercise such as walking or swimming, this could provide the gentlest total fitness system for you.

Alexander Technique

It's very likely that your joints have become stiff and your muscles have lost flexibility through years of bad posture. As time goes by, the body tends to settle into the position most frequently adopted during work or play. If your body has been forced to retain certain attitudes for long periods, it adapts to prevent strained muscles. It does this by toughening up the connective tissue that supports each muscle, which in turn fixes the body into a distorted shape. Continual movement keeps the connective tissue pliable. The Alexander Technique works on your balance, posture and movement to release tension and re-align the body correctly. A teacher works on a one-to-one basis, seeking out your distorted muscles and reorganising them through natural movement patterns. An average of twenty-five lessons are needed for full benefit.

Dance

Ballet, tap, jazz, flamenco, belly dancing – there are endless choices of dance classes, all of which combine the advantages of increasing flexibility, strengthening your muscles and giving your heart an aerobic workout. Ballet is particularly elegant, improving posture, strengthening your back and doing wonders for your legs, while flamenco really encourages you to present yourself proudly to the world. Never feel too self-conscious to join such classes. Everyone is hopeless to begin with, but progress is fast. If you haven't danced for years, a good class could really loosen up your inhibitions, while making you feel that you're mastering a new skill.

Body conditioning

This concentrates on stretching and strengthening all the muscle groups and could be for you if you like your exercise classes without frills. You'll need to combine it with an aerobic activity to work your cardiovascular system too.

Callanetics

These are basically isometric exercises. Callan Pickney claims to be able to make your body look ten years younger in ten hours. It's a tough programme that works the deep muscle groups to 'pull in and pull up' your body. The movements are minimal and precise, and certainly work fast to firm you up. The home video is particularly clear to follow, and you don't need much space to move about in. Callan claims that two hour-long sessions a week will slim hips, flatten your stomach, lift your bust and firm your thighs in a matter of weeks, then you only need to do a one-hour-a-week session to maintain your new figure. This is an excellent body-shaping programme that you can do at home, but you'll need to do flexibility exercises plus an aerobic workout to get a full fitness programme.

STRENGTH

Building up your muscles means you have to work them against resistance. The most efficient way to do this is with weight training, either by using free weights or with special machines at the gym such as Nautilus. Basically, fewer repetitions of an exercise with heavy weights builds muscle, whereas more repetitions with lighter weights shapes them. You need to do both sorts to work the muscle through its full length. This is the kind of exercise that can really change your shape. Fifteen minutes of weight training three times weekly is a good starting rate.

Weight training is best practised at a reputable gym, where all the best equipment will be on offer to you and you'll be given a lesson on how to use the machines. You'll also be shown how to use free weights, which you can then carry on using at home. Women usually start with three-to five-pound dumb-bells, building up as you gain strength. Weight training with free weights is particularly good for building and shaping the arms and chest area. For a home gym, combine these with an exercise bike to work your legs and give you a cardiovascular workout, plus a flexibility routine such as yoga, and you've got a good whole-body system.

AEROBIC FITNESS

Aerobic exercise is the best way to increase metabolism, burn up fat and strengthen your heart. This means exercising at low but prolonged intensity, to make the body draw on its fat reserves as fuel. High intensity short bursts of exercise are fuelled predominantly by blood glucose and then by glycogen, a carbohydrate stored in the liver and lean tissue. Exercising at a lower intensity for longer causes the body to spare its glucose and glycogen reserves, and to draw on fat. When you exercise hard enough and for long enough, stored fat pours out of your fat cells and begins to circulate in your bloodstream. Similarly sugar flows out of your liver, and this fat and sugar in your blood mimics the blood content after meals when the fat and sugar in your food are being circulated. This is sensed by the appetite centres in your brain, which then turn off their hunger signals, so exercise can act as an appetite suppressant.

To get this effect you'll need to work for thirty minutes at an intensity that gets your heart beating at 70 to 90 per cent of its maximum obtainable rate. To work out your maximum heart rate, subtract your age from 220, and then reduce this number by one quarter: so if you're forty a safe limit during exercise is 135 per minute. Then while you're exercising take your pulse at the side of your throat or inside your wrist for ten seconds, then multiply by six. Your beats per minute figure should be between 70 and 90 per cent of the rate you calculated above.

The best aerobic exercises are walking, jogging, swimming, stationary cycling and aerobic dancing. Walking, jogging and stationary cycling primarily benefit the legs, quickly producing visible changes in the calf and thigh muscles. Swimming is more of a total body workout, challenging all the major muscle groups. It particularly strengthens muscles in the arms, shoulders and back. Aerobic dancing can provide a total body workout if the routine is well balanced, varied and continuous.

THE GENTLEST, MOST EFFECTIVE PROGRAMME FOR FORTYSOMETHINGS

Walk or swim for half an hour three times a week, do a half hour stretching routine such as yoga on two other days, and do fifteen minutes of weight training on the other two days with hand weights. Bear in mind that your aerobic walking and swimming must keep your heart rate up to the desired level for any benefit to occur. This adds up to three hours of exercise a week. If you also do some gardening, go out dancing, run up the stairs and think about stretching your body whenever you can, plus consciously correct your posture, all-round fitness can be yours.

NINE

A - Z of Health and Therapies

The health issues that most affect you – and the therapies to meet
your needs.

ACUPUNCTURE

This is the most popular and effective healing technique offering drug-free pain relief. If you've been put off trying this therapy for fear of feeling like a human pin-cushion, the skill of a *registered* practitioner should make this a relaxed and pleasurable experience. True, Maggi once suffered a massive bruise on her inner knee from a painfully inserted needle, but this is rare. Originating in China, the classic theory goes that an invisible system of meridians links the various energies in the body. There are twelve main meridians, and blockages or imbalances can alter the flow of this *Chi* energy, resulting in illness. Stimulating the acupuncture points along the meridians restores the flow to normal.

Conventional doctors prefer to explain the phenomenal success of acupuncture by suggesting that the needles stimulate sensory nerves in the skin and muscles, and when these impulses reach the brain they block out pain signals through the release of endorphins.

Acupuncture is particularly effective for the relief of asthma, migraine, back pain, digestive disorders and PMT. It can also help in the control of emotional disturbances, stress and addictions such as smoking and alcohol.

Acupressure uses hard finger pressure instead of needles, and is a useful trick to learn as it can be self-administered. (Thus if you suddenly notice that someone you're talking to is pressing hard on some spot around their head, neck or hands, but their facial expression remains serene, you know that they are relieving the pain of your company in their own polite, inscrutable fashion.)

AROMATHERAPY

This two-thousand-year-old therapy from the Middle East is a most heady and exotic experience, basically involving some minion massaging your body from head to foot with aromatic unguents while you recline like an ancient Egyptian goddess. *Ergo*, it costs an equitable amount (but who is complaining?) for an hour of two of bliss. The essential oils used are extracted from plants, leaves, flowers, bark, roots, seeds, stalks and resins, and an enormous amount of plant material goes into making a few precious drops of oil. Massaged into the skin (diluted in a carrier oil such as almond or wheatgerm), added to the bath or directly inhaled, they can have remarkable results in healing wounds and scar tissue, the treatment of acne and other skin problems, nervous disorders such as migraines, anxiety and insomnia and medical problems such as rheumatism. Some swear it helps to shift cellulite, too. Some oils definitely have antiseptic powers, and are widely used in conventional treatments. Aromatherapists claim to be able to detoxify the body, boost the immune system, improve lymphatic drainage and balance the body's energies. Doctors explain the effect of scent on the body and nervous system this way: our sense of smell is triggered by airborne molecules landing for a few milliseconds on tiny receptors inside our noses. There are at least fifty different types of receptors and all smells affect a combination of them. These receptor nerve cells are connected to the limbic area of the brain – the region responsible for moods and emotions. So some perfumes make us happy, some randy, and some can make us feel physically sick. If you find a particular scent relaxing this starts a physiological response and you find yourself soothed.

Dr George Dodd at the University of Warwick has developed a small scented sponge for sufferers of anxiety attacks. Just take a sniff for the same effect as an instant shot of valium. He's now working on aromatic appetite suppressants. (So those eighteenth-century aristos with their nosegays had the right idea all along.)

Try these at home, added to the bath or massaged directly on to the skin:

For depression: frankincense, rose, bergamot, geranium, lavender.
Muscular aches and pains: rosemary, lavender.
To alleviate fatigue: ylang-ylang, sandalwood, patchouli, mandarin.
Anti-stress: jasmine, fennel, neroli, hyssop.
Digestive problems: peppermint.
Fluid retention: lemon, juniper, orange.

ARTHRITIS

Osteoarthritis is a common joint complaint, which results when the spongy cartilage of the joints grinds away, leaving the bones unpadded. Unhappily, the majority of people over forty show some evidence under X-ray of arthritic changes in some joints, especially in the fingers and spine, hips and knees. Persistent misuse of joints is a primary cause, so strenuous exercise should be practised carefully if sustained. Sportswomen and ballet dancers are at high risk, as are the very overweight, as this puts an extra burden on the hip and knee joints. To counteract, keep surrounding muscles strong with regular mild exercise, such as swimming, walking and yoga.

AUTOGENICS

This literally means 'generated from within' and consists of a series of mental and physical exercises designed to promote deep relaxation. The system needs to be taught, but once learnt can be practised almost anywhere, any time.

Developed by a German psychiatrist, Johannes H. Schultz, in the 1930s, this form of auto-suggestion aims at producing sensations of warmth and heaviness in the limbs, and regulates breathing and heart rate. Basically, this is it: in a quiet place, either lie on the floor or bed, or slump down in your chair. Close your eyes, and start by focusing on your arms. Repeat 'my arms are warm and heavy' several times, then move on through hands and fingers, and down the body through the legs and feet. Anywhere where you feel tension in your body, concentrate on warmth and heaviness seeping out of your muscles. Then think about your heart and say, 'my heartbeat is regular and calm'. You'll soon feel yourself relaxed enough to fall asleep, but if there's still work to be done cancel the session by clenching your hands and bringing them sharply up with a deep inhalation of breath. Then stretch your whole body and breathe out. The secret of success with this method is that it focuses you inward on the physical tension in your body, and while mentally involved with releasing it you are forced to stop worrying about outside issues. Thus you become more aware of how anxiety affects your posture and breathing.

BACH FLOWER REMEDIES

These days, the hippest drug to be on is Bach's Rescue Remedy, which, in basic terms, is the mere vibrations of Star of Bethlehem, cherry plum, rock rose and clematis transmitted to water by sunlight. The fact that this ethereal concoction is then taken preserved in brandy may have something to do with its sudden and mystical effect, but not for us to carp as it has got Maggi through many a sticky-palmed moment.

The devotees of Dr Edward Bach believe that the remedies treat emotional disorders rather than physical ones which are just a manifestation of trouble below. Dr Bach felt able to classify people into personality archetypes, each with a habitual negative emotional state, such as indecision or fear. He then, by some mystical divination, selected twelve plants as 'Healers' which would transform these states into positive ones, and discovered twenty-six more plant remedies to act as 'Helpers'. These are now available from many health food stores and homeopathic pharmacies. It can be a little disconcerting when consulting the list of negative emotional states to discover that you are suffering from all of them (self-disgust – crab apple; despondency – gentian; irrational thoughts – cherry plum; procrastination – hornbeam; etc,) and staggering out with the full range of thirty-nine little bottles. Should you do this, you could always pour them all together into a hip flask and slug them back in one hit, thus relieving yourself of all your negative emotional states and taking a crafty nip at the same time. Seriously though, two drops in a glass of water have been reported to have instant effects, especially in the case of panic or trauma due to accident.

BACKACHE

With four-hundred muscles and ligaments attached to the spine, it's hardly surprising that something gets strained from time to time, and four out of five people will suffer back pain at some time in their lives. Poor posture, badly designed chairs and beds, sudden injury or strain all can cause painful muscle spasm.

More serious is a damaged or worn disc bulging under pressure against the ligaments of the spine, which are very sensitive to pain. Speedy diagnosis and treatment are essential, as back pain can be the symptom of a number of diseases affecting the kidneys and reproductive organs. Once you have a diagnosis, decide whether your best option would be physiotherapy, osteopathy, chiropractic, Alexander Technique or rolfing.

A prolapsed ruptured disc may require surgery, so never have alternative treatment without conventional medical diagnosis. Hospitals offer physiotherapy, involving manipulation, massage, heat and traction, whereas osteopaths concentrate on realigning the whole body. Chiropractors offer similar techniques but tend to make direct adjustments to the spine. (See under relevant headings.) It is essential to go to a qualified practitioner.

To avoid back pain, be mindful of your posture, and always support the small of your back when sitting for long stretches. Check your bed by lying down on it and seeing if your hand fits snugly when inserted between the bed and the small of your back. The bed is too soft if you can't do this easily, and too hard if there's too much space. Always bend your knees when lifting things, and try not to carry a heavy shoulder bag on the same side all the time. Exercises such as swimming and yoga strengthen the back. When practising the Kama Sutra, be mindful of your lumbar regions!

For immediate relief from back pain, lie down with a hot water bottle held against the painful area.

BLOOD PRESSURE

The pressure of the blood in your circulatory system is a key indicator of the state of health of your heart, arteries and veins. Your blood pressure fluctuates all the time, due to physical exertion and agitation, but a measurement of 120/80 is considered ideal, although it normally increases with age, and in a healthy body blood pressure finds its equilibrium quickly. Continued high blood pressure puts a strain on the heart and kidneys, and can lead to a stroke or heart attack.

Stress, lack of exercise, excess weight and the birth control pill all increase vulnerability. So do smoking and a bad diet. Have your blood pressure checked annually after age forty.

BREAST CARE

As breasts have no muscle, but consist of fatty and glandular tissue, posture, pregnancy, dramatic loss or increase of weight and lack of support can all affect the size, firmness and shape of your breasts. The ligaments that connect the breasts to the chest wall can become stretched, and this is irreversible. However, exercising the muscles of the chest underneath and around the breasts can improve their appearance, so swimming, weight training and specific callisthenics are ideal. Good posture lifting up the ribcage maximises your assets. Lots of creams claim to firm the 'envelope' of skin encasing the breasts, but they are ruinously expensive and oily, and just brought us out in unpleasant rashes. Better to use your favourite body lotion massaged well in after the bath to keep skin supple and soft. Trials with Retin-A are currently underway to see if elasticity lost from connective tissue in the skin can be regained. Meanwhile, a well-fitting bra is still your best friend, alongside a healthy attitude regarding what your breasts are really *for*. Practically no one has perfect ones, let alone ones that match.

Examining your breasts regularly for lumps is the best preventative measure of all. One in twelve women develops breast cancer, but early treatment results in a high degree of success. Very few lumps are actually malignant, but early diagnosis gives you the greatest possible number of options regarding treatment, so don't hesitate a moment if you discover anything unusual. If there is a history of breast cancer in your family or you are over fifty, it is wise to have a mammograph (X-ray) every three years, as some abnormalities are too small to be felt in examination.

To examine your breasts

Choose a day soon after your period ends if you are pre-menopausal, as breasts change in density throughout the cycle. Stand in front of a mirror in a strong light and look carefully for puckering of the skin or discharge from the nipples. Raise your arms and check from side to side. Then lie down, and use the flat of your fingertips to press gently on the breast working in circular movements from the outside of the breast in towards the nipple. Check for any lumps along the collar bone and in the armpits. Report *any* changes from normal, as soon as possible.

CELLULITE

Although this condition is in no way detrimental to your health, and indeed was never even heard of until the French invented it about twenty years ago, it can cause more mental agony than many a medical complaint.

All sorts of pseudo-scientific claims have been made by cosmetic companies and beauty therapists about the causes of cellulite; some say it's a kind of fluid retention, others that your thighs are a kind of dumping ground for 'toxic waste' the body can't expel. Serious studies at Northwick Park Hospital in Harrow, Middlesex have shown that fat cells from cellulite-ridden areas contain no more water or toxic substances than other cells, just more fat. Nor is the connective tissue between these cells 'thickened' as is often claimed. Every living cell consumes nutrients and metabolises oxygen, and must excrete toxic waste products, but the fat cells on the thighs are no more toxic than fat cells anywhere else on the body. So why do women get cellulite and men don't, if the cause isn't hormonal either? It appears that fat cells in women are pouch-shaped and tend to group together in clusters, hence the ripple and bump effect where the body is fattest. Men's fat cells are long and thin, so they don't have the same problem.

So what can you do to get rid of this unsightly problem? Reducing your body fat through a low calorie diet is still your best option. As we age, we tend to store fat mostly in the lower body, so it can be harder to shift than when younger, but perseverance will achieve results. Building up the thigh and buttock muscles with exercise will help to tone up flabby thighs. If you feel you want to get rid of your toxins anyway, cut out processed foods, tea, coffee, alcohol and cigarettes, and increase your intake of fresh fruit and vegetables, and vitamins C, E and B.

Massaging your thighs with creams won't do you any harm either, but they won't 'eliminate tissue sludge' as many claim. A stiff massage with an astringent cream may temporarily pep up the circulation in the area, hence the popularity of strange green or gritty creams containing ivy, marine algae and all manner of exotic plant material. If buying an expensive cream gives you the motivation to pay your thighs some attention, by all means go ahead – there seems little point in spending twenty quid on a cream and then continuing to neglect diet and exercise. But don't bother with salon beauty treatments such as paraffin wax body wraps, faradic rejuvenators or deep heat 'Formostar' applications. These just waste time and money, plus you have to listen to the absolute drivel beauty therapists dish out as they try to blind you with science. You are not a moron, so refuse to be taken for one. Cellulite's fat, and that's that.

CERVICAL SMEARS

Cancer starts as a series of changes in the DNA of a single cell, which allow it to escape from normal growth controls and eventually spread to other parts of the body. Cervical cancer kills two thousand women a year in Britain, and it could be prevented by early detection. Five per cent of cervical cancers progress from a symptomless stage detectable only by smear, to an advanced invasive cancer in three years or less, so you really should *demand* a smear from your doctor every three years, and if you can afford to go privately, have one every year.

Smears detect any abnormal pre-cancerous or cancerous cells in the cervix. It's likely that a virus plays some part in the development of the disease, perhaps passed on sexually, as nuns rarely get it and prostitutes suffer the most. So the more sexually active you are with different partners, the more you need to be strict about your regular check-ups.

The best time to go for a smear is five days after the end of your period, as menstrual fluid can obscure cell irregularities.

Doctors at Glasgow's Beatson Institute led by Dr Saveria Campo are working on a new vaccine which may halt the virus thought to trigger the disease. Screening could identify the women who have the virus at an early stage, and an injection might clear them of the infection before it led to cancer.

Believers in holistic medicine have long been convinced that there is a link between personality and cancer. People who suppress their emotions while seething inside produce excess cortisol, a chemical released by the adrenal glands which gets rid of unwanted antibodies. But if too much cortisol is produced it mops up too many antibodies, leaving the body without adequate protection against infections, and possibly cancer. So when you're feeling really mad, let it all hang out. It could save your life.

CHILDBIRTH OVER FORTY

In California in 1956, a woman gave birth to a normal baby at the age of 57½, so should you be contemplating a baby over forty your body may still be ready and willing. True, your fertility begins to decline in your thirties, and the risks of birth defects increase, but the odds are still good. A woman of thirty runs a one in 885 risk of bearing a Down's syndrome child; this goes up to one in 365 by thirty-five, and one in one hundred at forty, but with the amniocentesis test (in which a little amniotic fluid is extracted from the womb and analysed for some sixty genetic abnormalities) the risk is not too great.

Before the days of the pill, it was quite common for women to carry on having children into their mid-forties. Often women would have a last baby and then their periods would just stop, bypassing the menopause altogether. Now births to older women are increasing again, reflecting the tendency of professional women to defer having a family for the sake of their careers, or the desire for children to cement second marriages. Today just over 1 per cent of women have babies in their forties. The actress Felicity Kendal had a child at forty-one, Farrah Fawcett at thirty-nine, Fay Weldon at forty-two. The writer says, 'To have a baby late you need health, money, love, friends and an equable nature.' It's actually believed that the older the mother, the higher the baby's IQ.

If you are hoping for another, or even a first baby over forty, have a talk with your doctor first. Your own health is perhaps the major issue – any medical conditions such as a thyroid disorder, diabetes or an ovarian cyst could make childbirth a dangerous enterprise. If your periods are regular, and you are in strapping good health, there's no reason why your pregnancy shouldn't be an easy one. Bear in mind that you will get much more tired than you did in your twenties, and the first couple of years with a new baby can be very gruelling, not to mention the effect it will have on your partner. But on balance, you may feel gaining another person to love is worth any short term sacrifices. Just be stringent about medical check-ups right from the start, and be realistic if you can about the risks. Ursula Andress, Goldie Hawn and Britt Ekland all had late babies, so why not you?

CHIROPRACTIC

Established at the end of the nineteenth century by Canadian Daniel David Palmer, chiropractic is more widely practised than any other form of complementary medicine, and has achieved remarkable results for backache sufferers. Chiropractors believe that manipulating bones and joints can relieve pressure against nerves causing pain, and cure specific structural problems affecting internal organs such as the heart and lungs. The spine is the centre of treatment, as displaced vertebrae cause a wide number of ailments. Some chiropractors use X-rays to make diagnosis. Although the majority of visitors go for relief from back pain, chiropractic is also effective in the treatment of other related problems such as migraine, asthma, constipation and menstrual disorders. The average course of treatment consists of six to ten visits at approximately £15 a time.

CRYSTALS

If you want to take a walk on the wilder side of alternative therapy, get yourself a crystal, the 'pet rock' of the 1990s. Hard core 'crystal channellers' believe that the lost world of Atlantis was powered by crystals, and Atlantians 'encoded' many crystals with information and teaching and put them on Earth. It sounds like harmless fun and sure makes pretty jewellery, although be warned, Liz Taylor's life is deemed to have fallen apart after she got all those big gemstones. The moral is, don't purchase more power than you can cope with. A crystal consultant will find the perfect one for you. If someone with bad vibes touches your stones you may have to have them cleared by a crystal cleaner (in California, where they're crazy for this sort of flapdoodle, they make house calls).

Once you have found your stone, you can programme your pet to try to achieve a certain task for you, as they are supposed to store information and generate energy. Amongst those who crystal gaze are Tina Turner, Goldie Hawn, Richard Gere and Oprah Winfrey. Try blue lace agate to relieve stress, white aragonite to purify your home, and black tourmaline to prevent psychic energy drain by other people.

DEPRESSION

Professor Hannah Steinberg at University College, London believes that people suffering from the milder forms of depression should try taking up some form of exercise before resorting to tranquillisers or anti-depressants. Light but sustained exercise brings about the release of endorphins in the body, chemicals which naturally make you feel better. Also the more physically fit you are, the more able to withstand mental stress.

Of course we all feel depressed at times, but fully-fledged depressive illness occurs when the symptoms are long-lasting. Psychotherapy through counselling or group therapy is the best treatment for clinical depression, so don't let your doctor fob you off with drugs if you think you are a sufferer. Changes in diet may also be necessary, as deficiencies in calcium, magnesium, vitamin B6 and the amino-acids can contribute to the problem. If someone you know seems very depressed, don't lose patience with them; they really need your sustained help through regularly expressed love and understanding. Having suffered from post-natal depression Maggi remembers the feelings of hopelessness and frustration. Life doesn't seem worth living, and being told to keep your chin up and cheer up just makes you feel more alienated by the seeming insensitivity of others. Depression is a form of illness and needs support. Doctors and friends are the only ones who can give it.

DIGESTION

Your stomach makes acid all the time, much needed for the digestion of food. But too much acid can be produced as the result of eating too much starchy or sugary food. Any backflow of acid from the stomach will creep up the oesophagus, causing a burning sensation behind the breastbone and difficulty in swallowing – this is known as heartburn. The pain can be severe enough to be mistaken for a heart attack, but with the latter there is usually accompanying perspiration, shortness of breath and shooting pains down the left arm. Bloating after meals is usually caused by gas – excessive air in the stomach or intestines, often the result of gulping food too quickly, anxiety, obesity or constipation.

A change of eating habits should put paid to most forms of indigestion –

that means cutting down on starch, sugar, spicy foods, alcohol and carbonated drinks. If symptoms persist you may have problems with your gall bladder or pancreas, and should consult a doctor.

FLOATATION TANKS

Floatation tanks were originally developed in the fifties by Dr John Lilly, a neurophysiologist who was investigating the results of depriving the body and mind of all external stimuli. Instead of being horribly unpleasant, self deprivation was found to inspire a deep sense of well-being and relaxation.

Tank facilities are springing up all over, as stressed-out high-flyers book up for regular sixty-minute sessions. The glass-fibre tanks measure eight and a half feet by four and a half by seven, and are filled with ten inches of an Epsom-salts-in-water solution. This gives a warm, dark and silent environment to float in, and all you have to do is empty your mind while all your troubles float away. Tests have shown reductions in heartbeat and blood pressure while floating, and in this state of deep relaxation you should feel more in touch with the secrets of your inner being and able to find solutions or inspiration to deal with your current hassles.

GINSENG

Amongst the claims for this extraordinary root are that regular use reduces the degenerative effects of ageing, revs up your libido, stabilises blood pressure, helps the body adapt to stress, corrects thyroid and adrenal dysfunction, and generally prevents infections. It is classified pharmacologically as an adaptogen.

The best ginseng in the world is Wild Asian, followed by Chinese red and Korean red. Amongst the goodies ginseng contains are vitamins A, B, B2, B3, B12, C and E; calcium, iron, phosphorus, starch, oestrogenic substances and saponin panaxin. The ideal dose is one or two grammes daily, for at least one month to feel any effects. No clinical trials have come up with any positive proof that this fleshy man-shaped root can deliver all its promises, and the fact that one tends to take such things while feeling low, then stop when feeling better, leaves its effects impossible to measure. But the Chinese swear by it and have done so for thousands of years.

HERBALISM

The history of herbalism has been surrounded by much myth and magic, but at least a third of the most powerful medicinal drugs used today come from plants. There are at least 350,000 known species of plants of which only about 10,000 have been tested medicinally, so it's not unfeasible that there's a cure for cancer growing peacefully somewhere, waiting to be discovered. Women have always had an affinity with plants and their uses, whether as cures, poisons or aids to childbirth, and fear of their power led to persecution and witch-burning in earlier centuries. These days many cosmetics have herbal additives as nature is in vogue again, and herbal teas treat numerous light ailments from indigestion to insomnia. What is strange is not that we are returning to herbal remedies, but that we ever lost faith in them in the first place. Inorganic chemical medicines are a very recent development, but drug companies are having difficulty finding new active ingredients and are turning back to plant substances again. Garlic clove oil kills off typhoid bacteria twenty-four times more effectively than carbolic acid, for example.

The extraordinary thing about plants is that alongside the medicinal substances, they also contain secondary enhancing or side-effect-eliminating substances, so it could be safer to take the leaf of a plant as a complete medicine than the curative substance extracted from the plant on its own.

Herbalists don't claim to cure diseases as such, but to return the body's balance to normal. Herbalists are not medically trained but do undergo several years' training, and he or she will arrive at a diagnosis by taking a detailed medical and dietary history of the patient. Each patient will receive a tailor-made herbal remedy designed to stimulate the body's own defences. The future of medicine may lie in the plant world, and making one's own cosmetics from herbal sources can result in a far more effective product than anything you can buy. Fascinating discoveries lie ahead.

HOMEOPATHY
This is a system of medicine based on the theory that 'like can cure like' – in other words, a substance which causes certain symptoms in a healthy person will also cure the same symptoms in a sick one, and the more diluted the drug, the more effective it becomes.

These days many fully qualified medical doctors also practise homeopathy. There are more than 2,000 remedies derived from plant, mineral or animal sources, and they come in the form of powders, pills, tinctures, ointments or granules.

Homeopathy was originally developed by a Leipzig physician, Dr Samuel Hahnemann, who found that taking cinchona bark gave him the same symptoms as malaria sufferers, and yet this same bark was being used to treat malaria. He proceeded to give small doses of the medicine to healthy people and noted the effects. Over the years he built up a list of substances and the symptoms they produced in healthy people, then treated sick patients with the same symptoms with the same drug. He also started to dilute the doses to eliminate side-effects. Doctors now give the smallest effective dose to patients, and some of these dilutions are so extreme that only a few molecules – or even none – of the original drug are left. In the latter case it is claimed that the original substance has imprinted itself on the water molecules.

Homeopathic remedies are believed to be effective for most reversible illnesses and acute infections, but not where surgery is needed. After treatment there may be a temporary increase in symptoms before the improvement starts. Homeopathic remedies can also be used as preventives and work well on animals.

HORMONE REPLACEMENT THERAPY

First a few words about oestrogen. As the ovaries start running out of eggs, the rate at which they produce oestrogen slows down and finally stops. As this happens, periods become more erratic, and finally cease, as no womb lining is forming to receive the eggs. The ovaries continue to manufacture androgen in the same amount as usual, and after menopause this androgen is converted into estrone (a weaker form of oestrogen) in a woman's fat cells. This explains why overweight women have more oestrogen than slimmer ones, but it is far weaker than pre-menopausal oestrogen, so symptoms of the change will eventually start.

HRT is actually oestrogen replacement, to alleviate all the unpleasant side-effects of the menopause. But taking oestrogen alone can increase the risks of cancer of the womb, so it is combined with progestogen (often called progesterone, which is synthetic), to balance the effects and cause a monthly bleed, so that oestrogen doesn't accumulate in the womb. If you have had your womb removed (hysterectomy), you'll only need the oestrogen. HRT will not be recommended at all if you have heart disease or a history of breast cancer.

The amounts of oestrogen and progestogen you are given should be carefully balanced so as to be right for your body. Prescribed by your doctor on the NHS, it is available in the following forms:

✹ *Tablets* – taken by mouth.

✹ *Creams* – placed in the vagina.

✹ *Patches* – the size of a 10p piece, they are stuck on the skin of the buttocks, and have to be changed twice a week.

✹ *Implants* – under the skin: these last three to four months.

HRT only works while you are taking it, so it's a long-term therapy. It's usual to take it for three years, then discontinue for a few months to see whether any symptoms remain. Women may take it for anything from five to fifteen years.

There is still some controversy over the safety of HRT. Showbiz personalities rave about it and declare it has helped them keep their good looks, while friends who have started it as early as forty say all their unpleasant symptoms of hot flushes, low libido and depression disappeared virtually overnight. Skin and hair bloom again, uncomfortable vaginal dryness disappears. But doctors are cautious about giving it a complete green light. One in five women don't seem to be able to tolerate HRT at all, experiencing worse side-effects than from the menopause itself.

Your best bet is to read up about it as much as you can, have a long talk with your doctor, and if he or she is unsympathetic or won't prescribe it, find another doctor who will. Make sure you are given the lowest possible doses to start with, and monitor your body carefully. Many women find the relief outweighs the risks, so it's up to you.

HYPNOTHERAPY

Hypnotherapists do not send their clients into deep trances from which they awake remembering nothing, but rather help them reach a level of deep relaxation from which they can be guided into the subconscious in order to come face to face with the initial cause of a problem. It's a state of heightened suggestibility, which can be achieved when the body is on the verge of sleep. Hypnosis seems to trigger a reduction of left brain activity which is logical, and an increase of right brain activity which is intuitive and imaginative.

Particularly helpful for those who want to give up smoking, hypnotherapy also works well on overeating, stress, phobias, obsessions, sexual problems and low self-esteem. It does so by helping to reveal to you the hidden memories, fears and unfortunate experiences that triggered the bad habit in the first place. The therapist will then feed you with positive self-imagery while you are in this highly suggestible state.

Hypnotherapists don't swing watch chains before your eyes or say anything along the lines of 'Now you are going into a deeeeeep sleeeeep . . .' They just talk in a quiet, slow and relaxed manner, asking you to think of peaceful images and keep your eyes on one fixed spot until they get tired. Afterwards you'll remember everything that was said, and you'll 'awake' feeling very refreshed. It can take as few as two or three sessions to quit smoking, six to eight for overeating.

MASSAGE

An expert massage is a luxurious treatment that can leave you feeling relaxed, pampered and zinging with mental and emotional well-being. All your aches and pains can be kneaded and smoothed away, and your skin and muscles will benefit from the improvement in blood circulation.

Just as we rub a pain better on a child, massage is both healing and therapeutic when administered to the whole body. Massage won't help you to lose weight or reshape your figure, but it could lead to a greater sense of body-love and awareness if you've been neglecting yourself. It can certainly help to improve bad posture, and through the aid it gives to lymph drainage, may help to alleviate fluid retention.

The massage should be given in a warm quiet room, on a table covered with towels.

Rolfing is a deep, manipulative form of massage which can be quite painful, but helps to realign the body. Invented by a doctor of biochemistry and physiology, Isa Rolf, it can counteract abnormal posture brought on by unhealthy modern lifestyles, which throws certain muscles into unnatural contraction, thus encouraging the connective tissues to thicken. By breaking down these thickened fibres, the body can be loosened and realigned. The treatment usually takes the form of ten one-hour sessions, the patient being photographed at regular intervals, so body changes can be monitored. Great pressure is exerted by the rolfer using knuckles, even elbows. It is also believed that we store emotional pain in hunched or contorted areas of the body, and releasing these kinks also releases the emotion, hence clients are encouraged to have a good cry if they feel the need. (Rolfers claim it's not the pain of their elbows that makes you want to do this, although it can approach torture at times. If it hurts you'll need more sessions to get properly loosened up.) People who have been rolfed get lasting results. One set of ten sessions can last years, if not a lifetime. You may find you grow half an inch to an inch in height, and feel greatly increased comfort and suppleness in your movements.

MEDITATION
Meditation needs be taught by an expert initially, but once you've grasped the mechanics, you can use this method anywhere, any time to lower your blood pressure, slow your heart rate and expel anxiety and depression. It can also help you to give up addictions, and cure asthma and allergies. At the very least it will always leave you refreshed and with renewed vitality.

Basically it's a way of shutting off your mind from all your daily preoccupations, and focusing on your quiet, inner self. It teaches you to calm your buzzing brain and helps you stay in control of your thoughts and emotions. Two fifteen-minute sessions a day should keep you relaxed and refreshed through even the most gruelling timetables.

To meditate, find a quiet place and sit in a comfortable position. (Lying down makes you too relaxed and liable to fall asleep.) Close your eyes and take several deep breaths. Consciously breathe out the tension in your body, working up from feet, legs, stomach and chest to shoulders, neck and arms. Then choose your mantra. 'Om' is a favourite Eastern one, or a word like 'peace' will do just as well. Concentrate on it and repeat it silently, slowly and rhythmically. If other thoughts pop into your head, as they surely will at first, just push them away with your out-breath and concentrate on your word. After ten to fifteen minutes, open your eyes slowly, stretch and get up. Aim towards twenty minutes with practice.

MENOPAUSE
The average age for the menopause is fifty, but many women go through it at forty, others as late as fifty-five. The medical definition of the menopause is the complete cessation of menstrual periods for twelve consecutive months, so you only know you've really been through it once it has passed. During the five to ten years before and after menstruation finally stops, a woman will experience many physiological changes, which vary in intensity from person to person.
These are:

Abnormal menstrual flow – either scantier or heavier by turns.

Sporadic periods – maybe missing two or three months at a time.

Hot flushes and night sweats – a rush of heat to chest, neck, face and arms, with quickening pulse and outbreak of perspiration. Flushes usually only last a few minutes, and can happen several times an hour. These occur when the ovaries secrete less oestrogen, causing the pituitary to react by secreting more hormones, sending the body's natural thermostat awry.

Insomnia

Headaches

Fluid retention

Mood swings

How can you calculate when your menopause is likely to occur? You can't really, but women who started menstruating early are likely to finish late as their fertility is high. Overweight women tend to have a later menopause, as do women who have children late. But there can be health risks with late menopause – breast cancer and endometrial cancer have been linked to the prolonged presence of high levels of oestrogen.

The menopause occurs when the ovaries stop producing oestrogen. If the ovaries have been removed by surgery, the menopause will follow. But if you have a hysterectomy but the ovaries are left intact, you will experience menopause at the normal time. Since menstruation started your ovaries responded to monthly instructions from the pituitary gland to produce an egg ready for fertilisation. Throughout the month the ovaries produce fluctuating amounts of oestrogen and progestogen. At menopause the ovaries ignore instructions from the pituitary and stop maturing the eggs (all the eggs you'll ever have are present in the ovaries since birth). After forty years and three hundred odd periods this stack of eggs is somewhat depleted anyway. The ovaries give up almost all hormone production, and as a result the lining of the womb doesn't form, so there is nothing to shed at the monthly period.

This decrease in oestrogen affects the bones, so you need to step up your intake of calcium. (See *osteoporosis*). You can do this by taking supplements and eating a diet rich in calcium – lots of skimmed milk, cheese, yoghourt, white bread, broccoli, cabbage and baked beans. Get plenty of exercise to keep bones strong, cut down on drinking and smoking, and keep on having plenty of sex. This should help you through what can be a difficult time. Many women actually feel better without so much oestrogen whizzing about. But others don't, and they may need Hormone Replacement Therapy.

OSTEOPATHY

The founder of modern osteopathy, Andrew Taylor Still, believed that faults in the musculo-skeletal system of the body were responsible for a wide variety of diseases. The spinal cord is the centre of the osteopath's attention, as this extension of the brain links to all the major organs of the body via the nervous system. Any interference with the spinal cord, through bad posture, injury or stress can affect the normal functions of major organs such as the heart, kidneys and liver. So as well as treating structural disorders of the joints and muscles, osteopathy may be used to treat asthma, headaches, digestive disorders and poor circulation. Treatment may consist of small rhythmical movements to stretch contracted tissues, gentle pressure and the movement of joints to take them through their normal range of mobility. This may result in alarming clicks, but it shouldn't be painful.

Osteopaths make their diagnoses by watching the way patients walk, stand and sit, taking medical histories and X-rays.

The massage, manipulation, stretching and moving of joints must be done with care, and should only be undertaken after the possibility of fracture, tumour or infection has been ruled out.

OSTEOPOROSIS

This literally means porous bones. After age thirty-five women start to lose their bone density at the rate of about 0.3 per cent a year, but after menopause this accelerates to near 1 per cent a year. Osteoporosis is defined as bone loss sufficient to cause fractures, as bones of the spine, wrist and hip become too thin to support their own weight and spontaneously break. This painful and disabling condition could be avoided by keeping up one's calcium intake from as early an age as possible, as 99 per cent of calcium in the body is stored in the bones and teeth where it provides bone structure and a calcium reservoir for the body. Bone undergoes constant rebuilding throughout life, and the hormone oestrogen is thought to slow the loss of calcium from the bones, and may help women absorb calcium. With the significant drop in oestrogen levels at menopause, brittle bones become a serious health hazard.

To protect yourself from later problems, attention to diet, exercise and the taking of calcium supplements is essential. Hormone Replacement Therapy at menopause to restore lost oestrogen also helps protect you. The Recommended Dietary Allowance (RDA) is 800mg of calcium a day for all adult women, 1000mg a day for women over thirty-five, and 1,500mg a day for post-menopausal women not on HRT. Milk is an excellent calcium source as it also contains vitamin D and lactose, both of which increase calcium absorption. One cup of skimmed milk has 300mg of calcium, an ounce of cheese around 200mg. Oily fish is another good source, as is yoghourt and fruit. Reduce your intake of phosphates as too much inhibits calcium absorption – these are mainly found in meat and as preservatives in processed foods. Stop smoking, as it is believed that nicotine impairs the activation of vitamin D in the liver, which in turn decreases calcium absorption. Cut down on caffeine, and build some weight-bearing exercise into your daily routine, as bones grow in proportion to the stress placed on them, which could be one reason why underweight women are at greater risk from brittle bones than plumper ones. Walking is the ideal exercise for bones, also running and biking if you're feeling more energetic.

PRE-MENSTRUAL SYNDROME

There are certain days every month when normal, sweet-tempered women suddenly feel like ripping their mother's throat out, running the car over their husband's face, or frying the children in the microwave. As we approach menopause and progestogen levels fall, the fog of misery that heralds the approach of a period seems to get worse. While regular periods are a reminder that you are still fertile with all the youth-giving hormones that entails, many women long for the menopause so that they can be done with the whole damn thing for ever. Meanwhile, there are plenty of ways to alleviate the symptoms.

Diet: Reduce sugar, processed foods, salt, wheat, carbohydrates, dairy produce, tea, coffee, alcohol and tobacco. Increase green salads and vegetables, protein and polyunsaturated oils such as sunflower oil. Take regular exercise.

Supplements: Take a multi-vitamin and mineral pill such as Optivite, A B complex vitamin and vitamin B6 in doses of 25 to 50mg every day, or 100mg B6 and 300mg magnesium for ten days before your period.

Evening Primrose Oil has shown remarkable results for some in relieving PMS. Take 2,000mg every day for ten days preceding menstruation.

Diuretics: See your doctor before taking these, then only use in moderation. Investigate some natural herbal diuretics available in health food shops.

Hormone treatment: Dydrogesterone is the most popular, taken in the form of pessaries. There are no side-effects and many women find this the most effective solution. See your doctor for a prescription.

REFLEXOLOGY

According to reflexologists, all the major glands, organs and nerves in the body have corresponding nerve endings in the toes and feet, and deep penetrating massage of these areas breaks up the crystalline deposits around these special nerve endings that cause illnesses. Thus foot massage can relieve tension, sinus problems, asthma, backache, poor circulation, haemorrhoids and even multiple sclerosis. Practised thousands of years ago by the Egyptians and the Chinese, scientific assessment of the curative power of this therapy has yet to be reached. Two forty-minute sessions a week for three weeks are generally recommended, but twenty or more visits may be necessary.

ROYAL JELLY

The Chinese take royal jelly very seriously indeed, believing it can slow down the effects of ageing on the immune system, inhibit the spread of cancer, and treat a wide range of ailments including arthritis, angina and psoriasis. At the very least it seems to work as a general tonic when you're feeling low.

The jelly is produced in the glands of worker bees and it provides the sole diet of the queen bee, creating phenomenal growth rate, fertility and lifespan. Whether it can do the same for humans remains unproven, and its exact chemical composition cannot be identified – but it does contain vitamin C, most of the B vitamins, all the amino-acids, six minerals, several enzymes, hormones and natural sugars. Tests have shown that the hydroxydecenoic acid contained in royal jelly, and not found anywhere else in nature, has an anti-bacterial quality which inhibits the development of tumours in mice.

If you've been ill, depressed or just get overtired, pampering yourself with a course of queen bee food could give you a lift. Always buy the fresh royal jelly, not the freeze-dried type, as the latter loses a lot of vital elements in the drying. Fresh royal jelly combined with honey in capsule or tonic form could have you buzzing with energy again.

SMOKING

Everybody knows why they should give up smoking these days. Alongside all the risks of cancer and heart disease, smoking also ruins your skin, causing it to age much faster. The nicotine and carbon monoxide in the smoke badly affect the circulation of the blood and oxygenation of the body tissues, causing hair and skin to look lifeless and dry. A substance called benzopyrene in cigarette smoke also uses up the body's supply of Vitamin C – and research has shown there is hardly any difference between the skin of a forty-year-old smoker and a non-smoker of seventy! The constriction of blood vessels in the face reflects the premature ageing and damage going on in the lungs, arteries and even your bones.

So how the hell are you going to stop? People don't smoke because they want to give themselves a terrible time; they smoke because they really like it. In fact they like almost everything about it – the lighters, the striking of matches, the first deep inhalation, even the overflowing ashtrays and smoke-filled rooms. Cigarettes are for when you feel bored, excited, nervous, calm, happy, depressed. A cigarette suits every occasion. As somebody once said, 'Lighting up a cigarette makes me feel like an abused women in a blues song.' They make you feel sophisticated, witty, weary and worldy-wise. Going outside with another smoker for a quick puff at a non-smokers' gathering leads to instant intimacy and a sense of shared sin. Smoking is romantic, sexy and sassy. It's great with a partner, and even better alone. So how the hell are you going to stop?

Because you know you've got to, don't you? You've got to stop behaving like you're acting opposite Humphrey Bogart all the time, and face facts. Many people actually wait until they're coughing up blood before they stop; many leave it too late. But the sinister mystique of smoking masks the fact that it's more than just another dirty habit like picking your nose. It can kill you in a horribly unattractive way.

A survey among friends who've kicked the killer weed reveals three methods that have worked. One is just stopping. To do this you have to catch the right moment in your life, or be convinced that you're so near death that you have no choice. Most people need more help than this. Method number two is slowly cutting down. This is a slow process and can lead to endless lapses. Maggi's brother and sister-in-law cut down from massive nicotine consumption to none in about a year by going through all the stages of cutting down, changing to lighter brands, using holders, chewing nicotine gum. They admit to still having the occasional craving. Number three method is hypnotherapy, and this seems to have the highest success rate. By replacing destructive behaviour patterns with their opposite, you can change your programming to a set of new instructions to nurture your body instead of trying to destroy it. If you're still smoking, you know it's only a matter of time. One of you is going to have to go. And once you've stopped, it's amazing how neurotic and unwholesome other people who still do it look.

STRESS

Working mothers with two or more children are probably the most stressed people on the planet. There are increasing stories in the news of women keeling over and going into comas because their bodies and brains cannot cope with *one more thing*. A woman's life is so jam-packed with stress triggers that we can often find ourselves in a perpetual state of arousal, and those two small glands which sit at the top of our kidneys are pumping out adrenaline day and night. We worry about children, work, money, home, husbands, lovers and friends. We want to do everything right and we want everyone to be happy. If something goes wrong – even if the cat is sick – we deem it to be all our own fault. We daren't show anger or emotion at work because it appears weak and unprofessional, and we don't admit the strain at home because everyone is looking to us for peace, comfort and love. Women follow unbelievable timetables in which they cook, shop in lunch-hours, clean and polish their homes, nurture children, hold down full time jobs, organise au pairs, visit in-laws, dance attendance on husbands and try to look perfect all at the same time. It's a miracle that we don't all crack up. Just having the job or the kids is stressful enough, and even a single woman with no one to worry about but herself has the stresses of modern living, noise, violence and crime to contend with.

So we all know why we're stressed. And we know how it feels – energy levels fall, chronic fatigue sets in. Headaches, skin rashes, muscular aches and insomnia, breathing problems, nausea and sweating are just the first stages. Stress hits you first in your weakest spot, and if the onslaught doesn't diminish, serious illness, particularly heart disease, can follow. If you feel tired and/or ill most of the time, some changes are going to have to be made.

The first obvious step is to cut out everything from your life that you really don't need to do. Delegate as much as you possibly can, and schedule some time into every day to relax away from the demands of everyone. Paying attention to your health is of paramount importance. Alcohol consumption often goes up in times of stress, but drinking is the very worst thing you can do. Better to practise deep breathing, get enough sleep, exercise regularly, meditate, take aromatic baths. Make sure you always eat well.

Your attitude to the stress in your life is probably the most important element of all. First you must stop denying your feelings. Venting them as they arise is the only way to dispel a build-up of tension.

Try to make some sense out of your life. People who handle stress well are those who find their lives meaningful and consistent, and that life's demands are worthy of commitment. A sense of optimism, of everything having a point, and an ability to accept negative emotions as normal marks out the stress-coper from the one who'll go under. Learn to say no, and try never to do anything you don't really want to do (banish *I should* from your vocabulary). If things have gone too far, seek help. Find a doctor who understands – you may need therapy, and you definitely don't need pills. What you must never do is press on regardless. It is thought that one of the main factors responsible for breast cancer is the withholding of emotion. Define your own needs and desires and make time for them – you alone are responsible for yourself, and you must learn when to put yourself first.

TRANQUILLISERS

The habit of taking the tablets starts insidiously. A crisis, a bereavement or a divorce may have you begging the doctor for something that will wrap your brain in cotton wool for a while. The numbness seems welcome after the pain. Benzodiazepines as found in valium, librium and ativan are the most commonly prescribed. In 1988 a government Committee on the Safety of Medicines issued a warning to doctors that these drugs should never be prescribed for a period longer than four weeks as they are highly addictive and can take years to get off again. They have many unpleasant side-effects such as anxiety, depression, sleeplessness and slowed reactions, and they don't cure anything – as soon as you stop taking them your nerves will be raw and easily stimulated, making you worse off than you were before. They can be harder to kick than heroin, so only accept them in cases of emergency, never for blunting everyday anxieties that stem from a more long term cause.

VARICOSE VEINS

Varicose veins can be unsightly and painful, and around 20 per cent of us suffer from them. They occur when blood from the larger veins found inside the leg muscles flows through connecting veins which contain small valves into the smaller superficial veins just below the skin's surface. The valves in a healthy vein work perfectly to allow the blood to flow back and forth between the larger and smaller veins, but sometimes these valves break down and as a result large volumes of blood start to flow into the superficial veins, distending them and making them knotted in appearance. The condition can be hereditary, but it is aggravated by overweight, pregnancy, an over-active thyroid gland, constipation and long hours of standing.

In more severe cases, iron from the blood may be deposited in the skin producing tattoo-like pigmentation, and eczema and ulcers are not uncommon.

Elevating the legs helps to relieve discomfort and swelling; weight loss through a high fibre diet and support stockings may also help. For more serious cases injection therapy may work – this involves the injection of a special fluid into the vein to disperse the blood and an elastic bandage is worn for three weeks. In the severest cases, surgery may be required to remove the damaged vein, followed by the wearing of compression bandages. Seek early help if you notice any change in your legs, and be cautious if ankles swell badly in hot weather. Rest the legs as much as possible, and if your job involves long hours of standing, try to keep moving or sit down as often as you can, with legs up on another chair.

TEN

Beauty Beyond

'Are you getting ready to be a sensational older woman?'

One of our culture's greatest misconceptions concerns what happens to women once they pass fifty. It's a conspiracy that has dogged women since the dim and distant Dark Ages, when women were merely regarded as walking wombs who became redundant after the menopause. Because men can go on producing sperm until they drop (who's muttering bloody typical?), fifty is no big deal for them. In fact if they have managed to amass some money and power, they can be seen as *more* exciting than younger contenders.

Thankfully this male/female imbalance is gradually evening out, and society is beginning to sit up and notice how much, if not more, older women have to offer.

Women of our mothers' generation mostly gave up on the quest for goddesshood over fifty, because they didn't want to be ridiculed or to shock. This is why Joan Collins is arguably the most important woman of the twentieth century. Single-handedly she has proved that a woman over fifty can be just as tacky, raunchy and sexually voracious as any younger Madonna. Our Joanie is always glamorous, always smiling, still carrying on with unsuitable men, and still an indispensable ingredient in the average dirty joke. If she could just polish up her repartee a little she could take the throne vacated by Mae West.

Where Joan Collins gets it right, Jane Fonda gets it wrong. Despite being as, if not more, beautiful, Jane has no humour and she tries too hard. One gets the impression that men just want to please Joan (and can't) while Jane just wants to please men. Over fifty a woman needs to be regal. Joan was recently photographed about to sweep into the Royal Enclosure at Ascot, when she was momentarily stopped in her tracks by a matronly steward who tried, unsuccessfully, to deny her access because she's not a royal. This same matron then had the nerve to say in the press, 'Why doesn't the silly woman act her age?' But that's exactly what Joan does. This sexagenarian potentate (sex-pot for short) *knows* that you've got to be over fifty and preferably sixty before you can *dare* to be totally outrageous.

Of course lots of women don't like Joan Collins much and have no intention of trying to emulate her. There are many other ways of being a sensational older woman.

You can choose to give up sex altogether (lots of women do so with relief) and become a Matron Saint. These women devote their lives to being truly useful and effective in the community, and can often be found furtively trying on petal hats like the Queen Mother's in department stores. They can be very glamorous too – Nancy Reagan with her anti-drugs campaigns, Liz Taylor with her work for AIDS and Jackie Onassis who just has to turn up anywhere to raise cash are all prime examples.

Best of all, you may feel most at home with the image of the Grande Dame – terrifying everyone with your steely gaze, your booming voice and your imperious stride. Echoing Queen Victoria, these ladies say in ringing tones, 'We are not interested in the possibilities of defeat, and we are definitely *not* amused.'

Grande Dames are very purposeful, very stylish, full of nerve and peculiarly English. Penelope Keith embodied the type in *To the Manor Born*. And they usually get the handsome hero in real life, too. They simply wither him into submission.

Germaine Greer is a personal favourite Grande Dame who can be a battle-axe or a bon vivant as the situation decrees. She is living proof that older women can and often do get the best of all possible worlds – they can be effective, sexy, strong and very funny all at the same time. They have an unswerving sense of themselves. What they want, they get. And they don't have to use feminine wiles to do it. They certainly wouldn't dream of having breast implants or ribs removed (Jane, are you listening) to get a man – or even to get a film part. Men are easy, and if they want film parts they start their own film companies, then ring up Willie Russell (*Shirley Valentine*) for a script. As Antonia Fraser says, 'The happiest women in the world are strong women.'

We really are the first generation who can expect to stay in the forefront of society until the end. After the menopause a woman still has a third of her life ahead of her, and we are the pioneering generation who are going into virtually unexplored territory. This is a truly revolutionary time to be middle-aged, for at no time in written history has a woman had such freedom and encouragement to carry on being exactly as she chooses.

Women's worst enemies are often other women. We tend to be very bitchy about famous women who put themselves up there to be judged. We still hang on to this downtrodden belief that women should be sweet, quiet, self-effacing and self-deprecating. Strong, noisy women are denigrated more by their own sex than by men. Our baser selves hate to see a woman going out and getting what she wants when we don't dare. If she keeps herself looking terrific we're envious of her self-esteem. We rake Joan Collins's face for wrinkles instead of admiring her immaculate skin. We almost *want* her to crumble suddenly, to prove that it can't really be done.

But it can. Katharine Hepburn is now in her eighties, and recently won an award for fashion. In her slacks, turtle-necks, trenchcoats and slouchy hats she still looks stylish and cool. 'If you just hang around long enough,' she says, 'people love you for it.'

But never mind the fighting talk, it really is an established fact that people over fifty enjoy themselves more than younger ones. A 1989 Mintel Report discovered that they are the happiest section of the population. And by the year 2000 one third of the total population of Great Britain will be over fifty, with 4 million over seventy-five. There will be fewer and fewer young people – right now the number of school leavers is dropping by 20 per cent.

This new older generation is like none other in history. They are better educated, more affluent, fitter and less prepared to take a back seat to the extravagances of youth. The media called them Woopies – Well-Off Older People. Unlike young working people with kids, jobs and high mortgages, they have time to spend on themselves and the money to do it, as pension and insurance schemes have matured and parents have died off leaving property.

The Mintel Report picture is overwhelmingly positive – older people go out more, spend more on clothes and holidays, and even start marrying again after a lull in their forties. They love their grandchildren, but are happy not to have the main responsibility for them. In America they have even built their own towns, leaving the violence of young urban lifestyles behind.

The only problems about being an older member of society will be staying fit and having enough money. So if you are forty now, start getting your act together today. There is much to look forward to in being of retirement age, but you really do have to plan ahead for it, just like the insurance salesman tries to tell you. If we're already losing our fascination with the young and naive, just think how much further society will have changed in your favour in another twenty years. To get the most out of it, start stashing away your cash and shaping up your flesh right now.

But enough of this heavy financial pestering – what you really want to know is how you're going to look, and what you're going to *wear*.

BEAUTY NOW WE'RE NINETY

Don't laugh, we're researching this one right now. What's for sure is that space-age surgery using lasers (no scarring), developments in anti-wrinkle creams of which Retin-A is just a forerunner, and possibly hormone therapy to combat hair loss, brittle bones and skin changes will all result in the kind of beauty treatments we can only dream about now. It's unlikely that we'll ever be able to extend our lifespans much beyond 120, because it would be very bad for humanity if we didn't make way for younger blood. Doctors believe there is a 'death hormone' that we are programmed to release at a certain age, to make sure we don't simply dodder on for ever. But at sixty you can expect to look like a woman in her forties if you absorb and utilize all the information in this book from now on.

Alongside staying fit, it's very important to continue looking sexy and alluring in your hairstyle, make-up and dress. This means eschewing those awful lacquered candyfloss hairstyles that older women adopt in the misguided belief they hide thinning hair. Better to keep your hair long, straight and unpermed, and wear it up in a French pleat. On some women long grey hair *can* look sexy, shiny and soft if it is constantly conditioned and kept a stranger to chemicals. Likewise blusher, lipstick and soft eye shading can give back colour and animation to the most faded complexion. Clothes should remain the same as you wore at forty. Elegant, flowing, soft, silky – anything so long as it's not uptight, buttoned-up, over-tweedy and shapeless. Just decide right now to perfect a look you can stay with for the rest of your life. You may have to lower your heel height a little and gradually show somewhat less skin, but lots of older ladies have sensational legs, elegant hands and regal necks which can still be shown off to much admiration.

To answer Byron's question, 'What is the worst of woes that wait on age? What stamps the wrinkle deeper on the brow?' we would answer that it's berks like him who can only equate beauty with youth. Everything is changing and moving forward all the time. It's up to us to shatter the myth of which is the best age for a woman to be. The best age is whatever you are right *now*.

Useful Addresses

The British Association of Psychotherapists
121 Hendon Lane, London N3 3PR – 081 346 1747

Eating Disorders Association
Sackville Place, 44 Magdalen Street, Norwich, Norfolk NR3 1UE – 0603 621414
(anorexia and bulimia)

The Institute of Complementary Medicine
21 Portland Place, London W1N 3AF – 071 636 9543

Women's National Cancer Control Campaign
1 South Audley Street, London W1Y 5DQ – 071 499 7532

The Women's Therapy Centre
6 Manor Gardens, London N7 6LA – 071 263 6200

The National Osteoporosis Society
Barton Meade House, PO Box 10, Radstock, Bath BA3 3YB – 0761 32472

TRANQUILISER ADDICTION
Tranx UK
081 861 2164 between 10 am and 4 pm if you wish to speak to a counsellor

Tranxline
PO Box 20, Liverpool L17 6DS – 051 709 5199

SCHLEROTHERAPY
Katherine Corbett
Second Floor, 21 South Molton Street, London W1Y 1DD – 071 629 2210

ELECTROLYSIS
The following organisations have rigorous training requirements for their
members, and they will send you a list of names and addresses on receipt of an
SAE: Mrs Edna Derbyshire, The Institute of Electrolysis, Lansdowne House,
251 Seymour Grove, Manchester M16 0DS (members have the letters DRE –
Diploma of Remedial Epilation – after their names).

Mrs Marylyn Ennever, British Association of Electrolysists, 3 Mersey Avenue,
Upminster, Essex RM14 1RA (members have BAE after their names).

ALTERNATIVE THERAPIES
ACUPUNCTURE
Lists of qualified acupuncturists from:

British Acupuncture Association
34 Alderney Street, London SW1V 4EU – 071 834 6229

Council for Complementary and Alternative Medicine
Suite 1, 19A Cavendish Square, London W1M 9AD– 071 409 1440
Publishes registers of qualified practitioners.

Register of Traditional Chinese Medicine
19 Trinity Road, London N2 8JJ – 081 883 8431

AROMATHERAPY
The International Federation of Aromatherapists
4 Eastmearn Road, West Dulwich, London SE21 8HA

CHIROPRACTIC
British Chiropractic Association
Premier House, 10 Greycoat Place, London SW1P 1SB – 071 222 8866

FLOATATION TANKS
The Floatation Tank Association UK.
3a Elms Crescent, London SW4 8QE – 071 350 1001

HOMEOPATHY
The British Homeopathic Association
27A Devonshire Street, London W1N 1RJ – 071 935 2163
Lists of medically qualified homeopaths

HORMONE REPLACEMENT THERAPY
The Amarant Trust
80 Lambeth Road, London SE1 7PW – 071 401 3855

HYPNOTHERAPY
Training College of Hypnotherapy and Counselling
10 Alexander Street, London W2 5NT – 071 727 2006

MENOPAUSE AND PMT TREATMENTS
The Women's Nutritional Advisory Service
PO Box 268, Hove, East Sussex BN3 1RW – 0273 771366

OSTEOPATHY
The General Council and Registrar of Naturopaths and Osteopaths
5 Netherhall Gardens, London NW3 5RR – 071 435 8728

The Devonshire Clinic
21 Devonshire Place, London W1 – 071 935 2565

The Hale Clinic
7 Park Crescent, London W1N 3HE – 071 631 0156
Offers full range of Alternative Therapies

Natureworks
16 Balderton Street, London W1Y 1TF – 071 355 4036
Comprehensive range of Complementary Medicine

EXERCISE TECHNIQUES

The Alexander Institute
16 Balderton Street, London W1Y 1TF – 071 408 2384

The Bloomsbury Alexander Centrre
80a Southampton Row, London WC1 – 071 404 5348

British T'ai Chi Ch'uan Association
7 Upper Wimpole Street, London W1 – 071 935 8444

The Feldenkrais Method
The Open Centre, 188 Old Street, London EC1 – 081 549 9583
or 0273 27406

Iyengar Yoga Institute
223a Randolph Avenue, London W9 – 071 624 3080

The Medau Society
8b Robson House, East Street, Epsom, Surrey KT17 1HH – 03727 29056

The Pilates Centre
Unit 1, Broadbent Close, 20-22 Highgate High Street, London N10 –
081 348 1442

Synergy Centre
1 Cadogan Gardens, London SW3 – 071 730 0720
(Pilates, Yoga, Avi Control).

British Wheel of Yoga
1 Hamilton Place, Baston Road, Sleaford, Lincolnshire NG34 7ES –
0529 306851

Overseas Addresses

AUSTRALIA
Acupuncture Association of Australia,
P.O. Box 1744,
Brisbane, Queensland 4001

Australian Chiropractors Association,
419 Victoria Street,
Brunswick,
Victoria 3056

International Yoga Teachers Association,
P.O. Box 207,
St. Ives, NSW 2075

Australian Osteopathic Association,
4 Coronation Street,
Geelong West,
Victoria 3218

Australian Institute of Homeopathy,
21 Bula Close,
Berowra Heights,
NSW 2082

CANADA
Acupuncture Foundation of Canada,
5 Roughfield Crescent,
Toronto, Ontario M1S 4K3

Canadian Chiropractic Association,
1396 Eglinton Avenue West,
Toronto, Ontario M6C 2E4

Canadian Institute of Stress,
Suite 3100,
3300 Bloor Street West,
Etobicoke, Ontario, M8X 2X3

Canadian Osteopathic Aid Society,
575 Waterloo Street,
London, Ontario N6B 2R2

Alcohol and Drug Dependency Information and Counselling Service,
Suite 2, 247 1/2 Portage Avenue,
Winnipeg, Manitoba R3J 0N6

NEW ZEALAND
Medical Council of New Zealand,
P.O. Box 9249
Courtenay Place, Wellington

Mental Health Foundation of New Zealand,
Box 37-438,
Parnell, Auckland 1

New Zealand Chiropractors Assocation Inc.
Box 2858,
Wellington

New Zealand Homeopathic Society Inc.
P.O. Box 67095,
Mount Eden, Auckland

SOUTH AFRICA
South African Medical and Dental Council,
P.O. Box 205,
Pretoria 0001

South African National Council on Alcoholism and Drug Dependence,
3rd Floor, Happiness House,
Cor. Wolmarans and Loveday Streets,
Johannesburg 2001

South African Acupuncture Association,
P.O. Box 583,
Parklands, 2121